Instant Workups:
A Clinical Guide to Medicine

Theodore X. O'Connell, M.D.
Kaiser Permanente Medical Center

SAUNDERS
ELSEVIER

1600 John F. Kennedy Blvd.
Ste 1800
Philadelphia, PA 19103-2899

INSTANT WORKUPS: A Clinical Guide To Medicine   ISBN: 978-1-1460-5296-8
Copyright © 2008 by Saunders, an imprint of Elsevier Inc.

Notice

Knowledge and best practice in this field are constantly changing. As new research and experience broaden our knowledge, changes in practice, treatment and drug therapy may become necessary or appropriate. Readers are advised to check the most current information provided (i) on procedures featured or (ii) by the manufacturer of each product to be administered, to verify the recommended dose or formula, the method and duration of administration, and contraindications. It is the responsibility of the practitioner, relying on their own experience and knowledge of the patient, to make diagnoses, to determine dosages and the best treatment for each individual patient, and to take all appropriate safety precautions. To the fullest extent of the law, neither the Publisher nor the Authors assumes any liability for any injury and/or damage to persons or property arising out of or related to any use of the material contained in this book.

The Publisher

Library of Congress Cataloging-in-Publication Data

O'Connell, Theodore X.
  Instant workups : a clinical guide to medicine / Theodore X. O'Connell. – 1st ed.
    p. ; cm.
  Includes bibliographical references.
  ISBN 978-1-4160-5296-8
1. Clinical medicine–Handbooks, manuals, etc.   I. Title.
[DNLM: 1. Clinical Medicine–Handbooks. WB 39 O18i 2008]
RC55.O26 2008
616–dc22   2008008620

Acquisitions Editor: Jim Merritt
Editorial Assistant: Greg Halbreich
Senior Production Manager: David Saltzberg
Design Direction: Lou Forgione

Working together to grow
libraries in developing countries
www.elsevier.com | www.bookaid.org | www.sabre.org

ELSEVIER   BOOK AID International   Sabre Foundation

Printed in China
Last digit is the print number: 9 8 7 6 5 4 3 2 1

About the Authors

Theodore X. O'Connell, M.D., is the Program Director of the Kaiser Permanente Woodland Hills Family Medicine Residency Program where he also directs the residency research curriculum. Dr. O'Connell is a partner in the Southern California Permanente Medical Group and an assistant clinical professor in the Department of Family Medicine at the David Geffen School of Medicine at UCLA. He is the recipient of numerous clinical, teaching, and research awards. Dr. O'Connell has been published widely as the author of textbook chapters, review books, journal articles, and editorials. He received his medical degree from the University of California, Los Angeles School of Medicine and completed a residency and chief residency at Santa Monica-UCLA Medical Center in Santa Monica, California.

Kathleen Dor, M.D., is the Associate Program Director of the Kaiser Permanente Woodland Hills Family Medicine Residency Program where she directs the maternal–child health curriculum. Dr. Dor is a partner in the Southern California Permanente Medical Group and a clinical instructor in the Department of Family Medicine at the David Geffen School of Medicine at UCLA. She received her medical degree from the University of California, Los Angeles School of Medicine and completed a residency and chief residency at Santa Monica-UCLA Medical Center.

For Ryan

You light up my life, little man.

Foreword

The first ideas for this text came from my experiences as a practicing clinician involved in resident and medical student education. Most medical textbooks are oriented on the basis of a known diagnosis. If one wants to learn more about congestive heart failure, hepatitis C, or bronchogenic carcinoma, traditional textbooks can be great sources of information.

However, patients do not come to the clinician labeled with a diagnosis, except for those problems which have been previously identified. Patients instead come with symptoms such as fatigue, edema, dyspnea, or memory loss. They may also present with laboratory abnormalities such as transaminase elevation, hyponatremia, leukocytosis, or hypercalcemia. It is the role of the busy clinician to utilize the history, physical examination, and selected laboratory or imaging studies to sort out the patient's present symptoms or laboratory abnormality and provide a diagnosis.

As I developed my clinical practice, I began creating a list of fairly standardized work-ups for common clinical problems. The work-up could then be tailored to each patient based upon history and physical exam findings. This process made it simpler for me to initiate work-ups, saved me time in ordering these tests, and helped prevent me from forgetting any important components of the work-up.

Over time, I found that many of our residents were carrying my work-ups in their pockets for use with their patients, and that colleagues began using them as well. I began adding background information so that it would be clear why each test was indicated and in which cases additional portions of the work-up may be appropriate. Then one day it hit me that there were many more symptoms and clinical problems that could be outlined and explained in a similar format. Furthermore, many other busy clinicians might like to use these quick work-ups to save them time in their medical practices.

This text is directed to primary care physicians, but may be beneficial for physicians in almost all specialties. The work-ups outlined in each chapter are suggested courses of action based upon the current medical literature. However, they are not a replacement for clinical judgment and may not be uniformly applied to all patients. Every patient is different, and the history and physical examination may indicate a need for more or less evaluation than my work-ups suggest. These work-ups should be viewed as general guidelines to help the busy clinician to be exacting and thorough while also being efficient. At the same time, deviating from these work-ups on the basis of clinical judgment is encouraged and expected.

I hope that this text eases your practice of medicine while helping you provide the highest quality care to your patients.

Derby Hospitals NHS Foundation Trust
Library and Knowledge Service

Table of Contents

General Discussion

Although there is no universal definition for acute renal failure, accepted diagnostic criteria include an increase in the serum creatinine level of 0.5 mg/dL if the baseline is less than 2.5 mg/dL, an increase in serum creatinine by more than 20% if the baseline is more than 2.5 mg/dL, a 50% decrease in the baseline calculated glomerular filtration rate (GFR), or the need for acute kidney replacement therapy. The GFR decreases over days to weeks in acute renal failure, and patients are often asymptomatic. Complete renal shutdown is present when the serum creatinine level rises by at least 0.5 mg/dL per day and the urine output is less than 400 mL per day.

False elevations of the serum creatinine can be seen with medications such as trimethoprim–sulfamethoxazole, cimetidine, and cephalosporins because these agents can inhibit the tubular secretion of creatinine without causing actual damage to the kidneys. However, these medications can also cause renal failure as a result of interstitial nephritis.

The causes of acute renal failure (ARF) can be broadly divided into three categories. The first is prerenal ARF, which is a reversible increase in serum creatinine and blood urea nitrogen (BUN) that results from decreased renal perfusion, leading to a reduction in the GFR. The second category is postrenal ARF, which is caused by an obstruction of the urinary collection system by either intrinsic or extrinsic masses. The third category is intrinsic ARF, in which the structures of the nephron are affected. This third category can be further subdivided on the basis of the structure that is affected: the glomeruli, tubules, interstitium, or vasculature.

Prerenal acute renal failure accounts for 60–70% of cases of acute renal failure. The major cause of intrinsic ARF is acute tubular necrosis (ATN), which is caused by an ischemic or nephrotoxic injury to the kidney.

It is always important to exclude a possible obstructive cause in a patient presenting with acute renal failure since prompt intervention may result in improvement or complete recovery of renal function. Bladder catheterization may be considered, especially in elderly men with unexplained ARF. Renal ultrasonography can be used to diagnose obstruction by assessing for hydronephrosis.

Probable causes of ARF may be identified from the history and physical examination. Urine collected before the initiation of intravenous fluid or diuretic treatment can be used to calculate the fractional excretion of sodium (FENa) using the following equation:

$$FENa = \frac{\text{Urine sodium/plasma sodium}}{\text{Urine creatinine/plasma creatinine}} \times 100$$

A FENa less than 1% suggests a prerenal cause of ARF. A FENa greater than 1% suggests an intrinsic cause of ARF, most commonly ATN. The FENa is often greater than 3% in intrinsic causes of ARF. It should be noted that a prerenal FENa of greater than 1% can occur in patients receiving chronic diuretic therapy or in patients with ARF superimposed on chronic renal failure. Conversely, an intrinsic FENa of less than 1% can occur with radiocontrast nephropathy and rhabdomyolysis.

Medications Associated with Acute Renal Failure

Prerenal Acute Renal Failure

- Angiotensin converting enzyme (ACE) inhibitors
- Angiotensin II receptor blockers
- Aspirin
- Cyclosporine
- Non-steroidal anti-inflammatory drugs (NSAIDs)
- Tacrolimus
- Prostaglandin inhibitors
- Radiocontrast agents

Intrinsic Acute Renal Failure

Interstitial

- Allopurinol
- Cephalosporins
- Cimetidine
- Ciprofloxacin
- Furosemide
- NSAIDs
- Penicillins
- Phenytoin
- Rifampin
- Sulfonamides
- Thiazide diuretics
- Trimethoprim-sulfamethoxazole

Tubular

- Acyclovir
- Aminoglycosides
- Amphotericin B
- ACE inhibitors
- Cisplatin

- Cyclosporine
- Foscarnet
- Ifosfamide
- NSAIDs
- Oxalic acid
- Pentamidine

Causes of Acute Renal Failure

Prerenal Acute Renal Failure

Dissection

Embolus

Heart failure

Hemorrhage

Intravascular volume depletion

- Diarrhea
- Diuretics
- Fever
- Insufficient fluid intake
- Sweating
- Third-space losses
- Vomiting

Liver failure

Massive pulmonary embolism

Medications

Nephrotic syndrome

Pericardial effusion with tamponade

Thrombosis

Intrinsic Acute Renal Failure

Glomerular

- Churg-Strauss syndrome
- Endocarditis
- Goodpasture's syndrome
- Henoch–Schönlein purpura
- Idiopathic crescentic glomerulonephritis
- IgA nephropathy
- Lupus nephritis
- Membranoproliferative glomerulonephritis

- Polyarteritis nodosa
- Postinfectious glomerulonephritis
- Rapidly progressive glomerulonephritis
- Wegener's granulomatosis

Interstitial

- Acute interstitial nephritis due to medications listed above
- Bacterial pyelonephritis

Tubular

- Acute falciparum malaria
- Cocaine
- Ethylene glycol ingestion
- Heavy metals
- Hemoglobin and myoglobin
- Incompatible blood transfusion
- Ischemia due to sepsis, shock, hemorrhage, trauma, or pancreatitis
- Medications
- Myeloma light chains
- Radiocontrast media
- Rhabdomyolysis
- Uric acid

Vascular

- Aortic disease
- Aortic dissection
- Atheroembolism secondary to atrial fibrillation
- Atheroembolism after procedures such as aortic catheterization, arteriography, or vascular surgery
- Atheroembolism after abdominal trauma
- HELLP syndrome
- Hemolytic uremic syndrome
- Malignant hypertension
- Postpartum acute renal failure
- Renal artery stenosis or thrombosis
- Scleroderma renal crisis
- Small vessel thrombosis
- Thrombotic thrombocytopenic purpura

Postrenal Acute Renal Failure

- Autonomic neuropathy
- Blood clots
- Catheter
- Crystals
- Prostatic hyperplasia
- Retroperitoneal fibrosis
- Stones
- Stricture
- Tumors (prostate cancer, lymphoma, carcinoma of the bladder, cervix, uterus, ovaries, or rectum)
- Valves

Key Historical Features

✓ Symptoms of heart failure (shortness of breath, fatigue, dyspnea on exertion, paroxysmal nocturnal dyspnea, orthopnea), which may cause decreased renal perfusion

✓ Pulmonary symptoms which may suggest pulmonary–renal syndrome or vasculitis

✓ Diarrhea or vomiting which predisposes to hypovolemia

✓ Abdominal pain suggestive of nephrolithiasis

✓ Benign prostatic hypertrophy symptoms

✓ Sinus symptoms which may suggest pulmonary–renal syndrome or vasculitis

✓ Bone pain suggestive of multiple myeloma or metastatic malignancy

✓ Trauma which may cause rhabdomyolysis

✓ Prolonged immobilization which may cause rhabdomyolysis

✓ Constitutional symptoms such as fever, weight loss, or anorexia which may suggest malignancy or vasculitis

✓ Past medical history, especially diabetes, multiple sclerosis, or cerebrovascular accident which may lead to neurogenic bladder

✓ Prosthetic heart valve or valvular disease as a risk factor for endocarditis

✓ Past surgical history, especially recent surgery and procedures that may increase the risk for atheroembolism, ischemia, or endocarditis

✓ Recent administration of contrast agent

✓   Medications

✓   History of intravenous drug as a risk factor for endocarditis

Key Physical Findings

✓   Temperature for evidence of fever/infection

✓   Blood pressure for hypertension or hypotension

✓   Head and neck exam for evidence of dehydration

✓   Cardiovascular exam for evidence of heart failure, heart murmur, or jugular venous distention

✓   Pulmonary exam for evidence of heart failure

✓   Abdominal exam, especially for evidence of bladder distention

✓   Skin exam for rash which may be a sign of interstitial nephritis, lupus erythematosus, vasculitis, thrombotic thrombocytopenic purpura, or atheroembolic disease. Splinter hemorrhages or Osler's nodes suggestive of endocarditis

✓   Extremity exam for edema

✓   Pelvic exam for masses

✓   Rectal exam for prostate enlargement or nodules

Suggested Work-Up

Renal ultrasonography	To evaluate for hydronephrosis as a marker for obstruction
BUN and creatinine (Cr)	To evaluate renal function BUN/Cr ratio >20:1 in prerenal causes BUN/Cr ratio 10:1 to 20:1 in intrinsic causes
Serum electrolytes	To evaluate for hyperkalemia. Serum sodium used to calculate the FENa
Serum glucose	Used to calculate serum osmolality
Calcium	To evaluate for malignancy
Phosphorus	To evaluate for phosphorus imbalance and possibly chronic renal failure
Albumin	To evaluate for liver disease or nephrotic syndrome

CBC with differential	To evaluate for infection, hemolysis, or thrombocytopenia
Serum osmolality	Used to calculate the osmolar gap
Urine dipstick and microscopy	Prerenal ARF may show hyaline casts
	Postrenal acute renal failure may show few hyaline casts or few red blood cells
	Acute tubular necrosis may show epithelial cells, muddy-brown, coarsely granular casts, white blood cells, or low-grade proteinuria
	Allergic interstitial nephritis may show white blood cells, red blood cells, epithelial cells, eosinophils, white blood cell casts, or low to moderate proteinuria
	Glomerulonephritis may show red blood cell casts, dysmorphic red cells, or moderate to severe proteinuria
Urine sodium level	<10 in prerenal causes of acute renal failure
	>20 in intrinsic causes of ARF
Urine creatinine level	Used to calculate the FENa
Urine osmolality	>500 in prerenal causes of ARF
	300 to 500 in intrinsic causes of ARF

Additional Work-Up

Creatine kinase	If rhabdomyolysis is suspected
Uric acid	If gouty nephropathy, malignancy or tumor lysis is suspected
PSA	If prostate cancer is suspected

Serum protein electrophoresis	If multiple myeloma is suspected
Complement levels	If lupus erythematosus, postinfectious glomerulonephritis, or subacute bacterial endocarditis is suspected (levels would be decreased in these conditions)
Antinuclear antibody	If autoimmune disease is suspected
Double-stranded DNA antibody	Elevated in systemic lupus erythematosus
Antineutrophilic cytoplasmic antibody	If Wegener's granulomatosis or polyarteritis nodosa is suspected
Antibasement membrane antibody	Positive in Goodpasture's syndrome
Antineutrophil cytoplasmic antibody	Positive in Wegener's granulomatosis
HIV	If HIV nephropathy is suspected
Antistreptolysin-O titer	Elevated in poststreptococcal glomerulonephritis
Serum haptoglobin, indirect bilirubin, lactate dehydrogenase	To evaluate for hemolysis if thrombotic thrombocytopenic purpura, hemolytic uremic syndrome, systemic lupus erythematosus, or other autoimmune diseases are suspected. Thrombocytopenia and schistocytes on peripheral smear are also seen.
Hemoglobin electrophoresis	If sickle cell nephropathy is suspected
Urine eosinophils	If allergic interstitial nephritis is suspected
Blood cultures	If endocarditis is suspected
Abdominal plain-film radiograph	If nephrolithiasis or ureterolithiasis is suspected
Abdominal/pelvic CT scan	If malignancy, nephrolithiasis, or ureterolithiasis is suspected
Renal biopsy	May be necessary to establish the diagnosis, determine the prognosis, or guide therapy

Laboratory test results consistent with acute renal failure (rise of 0.5 mg per dL or a 50 percent increase in creatinine above the baseline or a 50 percent decrease in the baseline calculated GFR)

↓

Medical history; current medications; review of systems to include systemic symptoms (fever, weight loss); and physical examination to include vital signs, heart, lung, abdominal, pelvic, rectal, and skin examinations

↓

Likely cause of acute renal failure apparent?

Yes   No

↓

Confirm diagnosis with appropriate tests. Diagnosis confirmed?

Yes   No

↓   ↓

Treat cause.   Electrolytes (plasma and urine)
                          Urinalysis with microscopic examination
                          FENa
                          Renal ultrasound

Prerenal	Intrarenal	Postrenal
BUN to creatinine ratio > 20:1	BUN to creatinine ratio 10:1 to 20:1	Ultrasound shows hydronephrosis.
FENa < 1 percent	FENa > 1	Serum and urine tests have similar results to intrarenal causes.
Urine specific gravity > 1:020	Urine specific gravity 1:010 to 1:020	
Hyaline casts in urine sediment	Tubular or granular casts in urine	
No evidence of obstruction	Ultrasound showing medical kidney disease or normal, no obstruction	
No evidence of intrarenal causes of acute renal failure		

↓   ↓   ↓

Hydrate.	CBC, ESR	Order CT (without contrast) if cause of obstruction is not evident.
Eliminate toxins.	Consider nephrology consult/ kidney biopsy.	Relieve obstruction.
Treat causes.	Eliminate toxins.	Consider urology consult.
	Treat causes.	

Figure 1-1. Algorithm for the initial evaluation of acute renal failure. (GFR = glomerular filtration rate; FENa = fractional excretion of sodium; BUN = blood urea nitrogen; CBC = complete blood count; ESR = erythrocyte sedimentation rate; CT = computed tomography.)

Further reading

Agrawal M, Swartz R. Acute renal failure. American Family Physician 2000;61: 2077–2088.

Albright RC Jr. Acute renal failure: a practical update. Mayo Clinic Proceedings 2001;76: 67–74.

Dursun B, Edelstein CL. Acute renal failure. American Journal of Kidney Diseases 2005; 45: 614–618.

Lameire N. The pathophysiology of acute renal failure. Critical Care Clinics 2005;1: 197–200.

Needham E. Management of acute renal failure. American Family Physician 2005;
  72: 1739–1746.

Pascual J, Liano F, Ortuno J. The elderly patient with acute renal failure. Journal of the American
  Society of Nephrology 1995;6: 144–153.

Thadhani R, Pascual M, Bonventre JV. Acute renal failure. New England Journal of Medicine
  1996;334: 1448–1460.

General Discussion

Adrenal masses may be discovered incidentally on abdominal CT scans and ultrasounds. The vast majority of these lesions are benign and do not require referral or treatment. The two most important factors in the diagnostic evaluation are the lesion's size and functional status. Lesions larger than 6 cm in greatest diameter are more likely to be malignant.

To determine the functional status of an adrenal mass, the patient should be assessed for signs and symptoms of Cushing's syndrome, pheochromocytoma, and hyperaldosteronism. These signs and symptoms are outlined below.

The differential diagnosis of incidental adrenal mass, in descending order of frequency, includes adenoma, metastatic cancer, adrenal cancer, cyst, pheochromocytoma, hyperplasia, lipoma, and myelolipoma.

If the adrenal mass is less than 3 cm, the patient has no signs or symptoms, and the screening laboratory tests noted below are normal, the patient should have a repeat CT scan or ultrasound in 3 months and then every 6 months for 2 years. If the patient has signs or symptoms or the laboratory tests are not normal, referral to a surgeon is indicated.

If the adrenal mass is 3–6 cm in size, magnetic resonance imaging (MRI) should be obtained and endocrine referral should be made.

If the adrenal mass is more than 6 cm in largest diameter, surgical evaluation should be obtained.

Any patient with a history of malignancy who is found to have an adrenal mass should probably have a needle biopsy of the adrenal lesion since metastatic disease is the most likely cause of the adrenal lesion in this situation.

Signs and Symptoms of Systemic Disease

Cushing's syndrome

- Abdominal striae
- Buffalo hump
- Diabetes
- Diaphoresis
- Easy bruising
- Hirsutism
- Hypertension
- Menstrual abnormalities
- Moon-shaped facies

- Obesity, especially central
- Osteoporosis
- Proximal muscle weakness
- Thin skin

Pheochromocytoma

- Headache
- Palpitations
- Paroxysmal hypertension
- Sweating

Hyperaldosteronism

- Hypernatremia
- Hypertension
- Hypokalemia

Suggested Work-Up

24-hour urinary metanephrine, vanillylmandelic acid, and pheochromocytoma	Used to screen for catecholamines
Plasma catecholamines	Some investigators suggest using plasma catecholamines to screen for pheochromocytoma
24-hour urinary free cortisol	Screening test for Cushing's syndrome
Serum potassium level, plasma aldosterone, and plasma renin activity	Screening tests for hyperaldosteronism in the patient with hypertension

Additional Evaluation

Dexamethasone suppression test is warranted if Cushing's syndrome is suspected and the 24-hour urinary free cortisol measurement is equivocal.

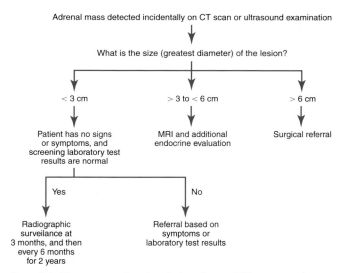

Figure 2-1. Management of incidental adrenal mass. (CT = computed tomographic scanning; MRI = magnetic resonance imaging.)

Further reading

Cook DM, Loriaux DL. The incidental adrenal mass. American Journal of Medicine 1996; 101: 88–94.

Copeland PM. The incidentally discovered adrenal mass. Annals of Surgery 1984;199: 116–122.

Higgins JC, Fitzgerald JM. Evaluation of incidental renal and adrenal masses. American Family Physician 2001;63:288–291.

Prinz RA, Brooks MH, Churchill R, et al. Incidental asymptomatic adrenal masses detected by computed tomographic scanning. Is operation required? Journal of the American Medical Association 1982;248: 701–704.

Ross NS, Aron DC. Hormonal evaluation of the patient with an incidentally discovered adrenal mass. New England Journal of Medicine 1990;323: 1401–1405.

Scott HW Jr, ed. Surgery of the adrenal glands. Philadelphia: JB Lippincott; 1990.

Vaughan ED. Diseases of the adrenal gland. Medical Clinics of North America 2004; 88: 443–466.

General Discussion

Primary amenorrhea is defined as the absence of menses by 16 years of age in the presence of normal growth and secondary sexual characteristics or lack of menses by 14 years of age in the absence of secondary sexual characteristics. In the classification of primary amenorrhea, hypogonadism refers to gonads that are not functioning and is associated with a hypoestrogenic state. Eugonadism refers to gonads that maintain normal steroidogenesis and is associated with a well-estrogenized state. An evaluation of breast development can be used to determine a patient's estrogen status. The pelvic examination then further narrows the potential causes by determining the presence or absence of a normal mullerian system.

The most common cause of primary amenorrhea is primary ovarian failure due to gonadal dysgenesis, most commonly as a result of Turner's syndrome. The second most common cause of primary amenorrhea is congenital absence of the uterus and vagina (CAUV), followed by idiopathic hypogonadotropic hypogonadism (IHH). Eating disorders such as anorexia and bulimia have the highest incidence during the adolescent years. Anorexia nervosa has a prevalence of 1% in the United States. The Female Athlete Triad overlaps with eating disorders and is characterized by disordered eating, osteoporosis or osteopenia, and amenorrhea in the setting of excessive exercise.

The first step in the evaluation of primary amenorrhea is a history and physical examination. If secondary sexual characteristics are not present, FSH and LH levels should be measured. FSH and LH <5 IU/L indicates hypogonadotropic hypogonadism. If FSH is >20 IU/L and LH >40 IU/L, hypergonadotropic hypogonadism is present. If hypergonadotropic hypogonadism is present, karyotype analysis is indicated.

If secondary sexual characteristics are present, ultrasonography of the uterus should be performed. If the uterus is absent or abnormal, karyotype analysis is indicated. If the uterus is present and normal, the patient should be examined for evidence of an outflow obstruction.

Medications Associated with Amenorrhea

Butyrophenones

Contraceptive medications

Divalproex

Domperidone

Haloperidol

H_2 blockers

Methyldopa

Metoclopramide

Opiates

Phenothiazine

Psychotropic medications

Reserpine

Risperdone

Sulpiride

Verapamil

Causes of Primary Amenorrhea

Eugonadism

- Androgen insensitivity
- CAUV
- Cervical atresia
- Imperforate hymen
- Polycystic ovarian syndrome
- Transverse vaginal septum
- 17-ketoreductase deficiency

Hypergonadotropic hypogonadism

- Ovarian failure (due to chromosomal abnormality, previous radiation, or previous chemotherapy)
- Pseudo-ovarian failure
- Turner's syndrome
- 46,XX gonadal dysgenesis
- 46,XY gonadal dysgenesis

Hypogonadic hypogonadism

- Congenital adrenal hyperplasia
- Congenital CNS defects
- Constitutional delay
- Craniopharyngioma
- Cushing's syndrome
- Diabetes (poorly controlled)
- Eating disorders (anorexia nervosa and bulimia nervosa)
- Hyperprolactinemia
- Hypopituitarism
- Hypothyroidism

- IHH
- Isolated gonadotrophin-releasing hormone (GnRH) deficiency
- Juvenile rheumatoid arthritis
- Malabsorptive bowel disease
- Malignant tumor
- Marijuana use
- Pituitary adenoma (prolactinoma)
- Pseudohypoparathyroidism
- Psychological stress
- Systemic disorders

Key Historical Features

✓ Menarche and menstrual history

✓ Sexual history

✓ Diet history

✓ Physical activity

✓ Past medical history, including history of chemotherapy or radiation

✓ Past surgical history

✓ Medications

✓ Family history, especially of infertility, genetic defects, and menstrual disorders

✓ Symptoms of hyperthyroidism or hypothyroidism

✓ Acne or hirsutism

✓ Headache or visual disturbances

✓ Anosmia or galactorrhea

✓ Cyclic abdominal pain

✓ Breast changes

✓ Easy bruising

Key Physical Findings

✓ Vital signs

✓ Height and weight compared against normative data

✓ Body mass index

✓ Evaluation of breast development

✓ Tanner staging to assess pubertal development

✓ Signs of an eating disorder such as parotid gland enlargement, Russell's sign, or dental erosions

✓ Thyroid examination

✓ Abdominal examination for masses

✓ Pelvic examination for inperforate hymen, transverse vaginal septum, clitoral hypertrophy, or undescended testes

✓ Rectal examination for skin tags, fissures, or occult blood that may indicate inflammatory bowel disease

✓ Evaluation for striae, buffalo hump, central obesity, or proximal muscle weakness

Suggested Work-Up

Pregnancy test	To rule out pregnancy
Serum FSH and LH	Should be measured if secondary sexual characteristics are not present.
	FSH >30 to 40 IU/L is suggestive of premature ovarian failure
	LH is more suppressed than FSH when amenorrhea is due to suppression of the hypothalamic–pituitary–ovarian axis
Prolactin level	To evaluate for hyperprolactinemia
Ultrasound of the uterus	Should be performed if primary amenorrhea is present and secondary sexual characteristics are also present
	If the uterus is absent or abnormal, karyotype analysis should be performed
	If the uterus is present and normal, patient should be evaluated for evidence of outflow obstruction

Additional Work-Up

Karyotype analysis	If persistently elevated FSH is found, karyotype is required to evaluate for a chromosomal abnormality

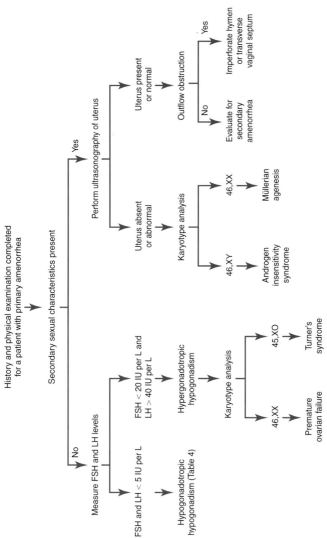

Figure 3-1. Algorithm for the evaluation of primary amenorrhea. (FSH = follicle-stimulating hormone; LH = luteinizing hormone.)

CBC, ESR, TSH, liver function tests, electrolytes, BUN, creatinine, blood glucose and urinalysis	If pubertal delay is present or systemic illness is suspected
Serum estradiol	To confirm hypoestrogenism if premature ovarian failure is suspected
Serum testosterone and dehydroepiandrosterone sulfate (DHEAS)	To evaluate for hyperandrogenism if signs of androgen excess are present
MRI of the sella turcica	If pituitary tumor is suspected
Radiograph of the hand and wrist	If short stature is present to clarify skeletal maturation for chronologic age

Further reading

Adams-Hillard PJ, Deitch HR. Menstrual disorders in the college age female. Pediatric Clinics of North America 2005; 52:179–197.

Kazis K, Iglesias E. The female athlete triad. Adolescent Medicine 2003; 14:87–95.

Master-Hunter T, Heiman DL. Amenorrhea: evaluation and treatment. American Family Physician 2006; 73:1374–1382.

Pletcher JR, Slap GB. Menstrual disorders: amenorrhea. Pediatric Clinics of North America 1999; 46:505–518.

Timmreck LS, Reindollar RH. Contemporary issues in primary amenorrhea. Obstetrics and Gynecology Clinics 2003; 30:287–302.

Warren MP. Evaluation of secondary amenorrhea. Journal of Clinical Endocrinology and Metabolism 1996; 81:437–442.

General Discussion

Secondary amenorrhea is the absence of menses for 3 months in women with previously normal menstruation or for 9 months in women with previous oligomenorrhea. Secondary amenorrhea is more common than primary amenorrhea. The most common cause of secondary amenorrhea is pregnancy. In addition to pregnancy, thyroid disease and hyperprolactinemia are also common causes of secondary amenorrhea.

Once pregnancy, thyroid disease, and hyperprolactinemia are ruled out as potential causes, the remaining causes of secondary amenorrhea are classified as eugonadotropic amenorrhea, hypogonadotropic hypogonadism, and hypergonadotropic hypogonadism. Outflow tract obstruction and hyperandrogenic chronic anovulation are two common causes of eugonadotropic amenorrhea. Polycystic ovary syndrome (PCOS) is the most common cause of hyperandrogenic chronic anovulation.

Clinically, it is helpful to separate patients who have secondary amenorrhea into those with and without hirsutism or signs of androgen excess. This can be done by history and physical examination as well as by laboratory studies. Physical examination may reveal hirsutism, acanthosis nigricans, acne, or clitoromegaly.

Medications Associated with Amenorrhea

Butyrophenones

Contraceptive medications

Divalproex

Domperidone

Haloperidol

H_2 blockers

Methyldopa

Metoclopramide

Opiates

Phenothiazine

Psychotropic medications

Reserpine

Risperdone

Sulpiride

Verapamil

Causes of Secondary Amenorrhea

Eugonadism

- Acromegaly
- Androgen-secreting tumor
- Asherman's syndrome
- Cervical stenosis
- Congenital adrenal hyperplasia
- Cushing's disease
- Exogenous androgens (anabolic steroids)
- Hyperprolactinemia
- Ovarian stromal hypertrophy
- Polycystic ovary syndrome
- Pregnancy
- Thyroid disease

Hypergonadotropic hypogonadism

- Postmenopausal ovarian failure
- Premature ovarian failure

Hypogonadotropic hypogonadism

- Anorexia nervosa
- Bulimia nervosa
- Celiac disease
- Central nervous system tumor
- Chronic liver disease
- Chronic renal insufficiency
- Cranial radiation
- Cystic fibrosis
- Depression
- Diabetes mellitus
- Excessive exercise
- HIV
- Immunodeficiency
- Inflammatory bowel disease
- Marijuana use
- Psychological stress
- Renal disease
- Sickle cell disease
- Thalassemia major
- Thyroid disease

Key Historical Features

✓ Menarche and menstrual history

✓ Sexual history

✓ Diet history

✓ Physical activity

✓ Past medical history, including history of chemotherapy or radiation

✓ Past surgical history

✓ Medications

✓ Family history, especially of infertility, genetic defects, and menstrual disorders

✓ Symptoms of hyperthyroidism or hypothyroidism

✓ Acne or hirsutism

✓ Headache or visual disturbances

✓ Anosmia or galactorrhea

✓ Cyclic abdominal pain

✓ Breast changes

✓ Easy bruising

Key Physical Findings

✓ Vital signs

✓ Height and weight compared against normative data

✓ Body mass index

✓ Evaluation of breast development

✓ Tanner staging to assess pubertal development

✓ Sings of an eating disorder such as parotid gland enlargement, Russell's sign, or dental erosions

✓ Thyroid examination

✓ Abdominal examination for masses

✓ Pelvic examination for imperforate hymen, transverse vaginal septum, clitoral hypertrophy, or undescended testes

✓ Rectal examination for skin tags, fissures, or occult blood that may indicate inflammatory bowel disease

✓ Evaluation for striae, buffalo hump, central obesity, or proximal muscle weakness

Suggested Work-Up

Pregnancy test | To evaluate for pregnancy

Prolactin level | To evaluate for hyperprolactinemia

TSH | To evaluate for subclinical hypothyroidism

LH and FSH | If PCOS is suspected (LH/FSH ratio may be elevated)

Additional Work-Up

Progestogen challenge test | If prolactin and TSH levels are normal, progestogen challenge is used to help evaluate for a patent outflow tract. A negative progestogen challenge test indicates an outflow tract abnormality or inadequate estrogenization

Estrogen/progestogen challenge test | Used to differentiate abnormal outflow tract from inadequate estrogenization. A negative estrogen/progestogen challenge usually indicates an outflow tract obstruction. A positive challenge indicates an abnormality within the hypothalamic–pituitary–ovarian axis

Testosterone and dehydroepiandrosterone sulfate (DHEAS) tumors | If signs of androgen excess are present to evaluate for adrenal disease and androgen-secreting ovarian

Estradiol level | To confirm hypoestrogenism if premature ovarian failure is suspected

17-hydroxyprogesterone measurement before and after ACTH injection | If adult-onset congenital adrenal hyperplasia is suspected

Urinary free cortisol and serum electrolytes | If Addison's disease is suspected clinically in the setting of premature ovarian failure

MRI of the sella turcica | To evaluate for pituitary tumor if the prolactin level is >100 ng/mL

Hysterosalpingography, hysteroscopy, or sonohysterography | If Asherman's syndrome is suspected in the setting of outflow tract obstruction

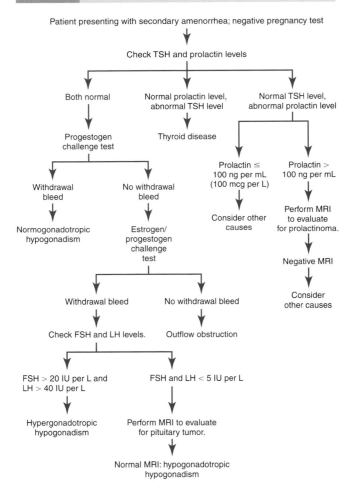

Figure 4-1. Algorithm for the evaluation of secondary amenorrhea. (TSH = thyroid-stimulating hormone; MRI = magnetic resonance imaging; FSH = follicle-stimulating hormone; LH = luteinizing hormone.)

Further reading

Adams-Hillard PJ, Deitch HR. Menstrual disorders in the college age female. Pediatric Clinics of North America 2005;52: 179–197.

Kazis K, Iglesias E. The female athlete triad. Adolescent Medicine 2003;14: 87–95.

Kiningham RB, Apgar BS, Schwenk TL. Evaluation of amenorrhea. American Family Physician 1996;53: 1185–1194.

Master-Hunter T, Heiman DL. Amenorrhea: evaluation and treatment. American Family Physician 2006;73: 1374–1382.

Pickett CA. Diagnosis and management of pituitary tumors: recent advances. Primary Care 2003;30: 765–789.

Pletcher JR, Slap GB. Menstrual disorders: amenorrhea. Pediatric Clinics of North America 1999;46: 505–518.

Speroff L, Fritz MA. Amenorrhea. In: Clinical gynecologic endocrinology and infertility, 7th ed. Philadelphia, PA: Lippincott Williams & Wilkins; 2005:401–464.

Warren MP. Evaluation of secondary amenorrhea. Journal of Clinical Endocrinology and Metabolism 1996;81: 437–442.

General Discussion

Anemia is defined as a decrease in hemoglobin or hematocrit level from an individual's baseline value. In general, normal hemoglobin levels are 1 to 2 g/dL lower in women and African-American men than in white men.

The initial laboratory evaluation of anemia should include a complete blood count, red blood cell indices, a reticulocyte count, and peripheral blood smear. The mean corpuscular volume (MCV) is used first to classify the anemic process as microcytic, normocytic, or macrocytic.

Microcytic Anemia

The evaluation of microcytic anemia begins by ruling out iron deficiency anemia. The definitive test for iron deficiency anemia is the serum ferritin, as a low serum ferritin level is diagnostic of an iron-depleted state. Other iron studies such as serum iron, total iron-binding capacity, and transferring saturation do not accurately distinguish iron deficiency anemia from anemia of chronic disease. In equivocal cases, a finite treatment trial with iron supplementation may help distinguish the two.

Other clues may help diagnose iron deficiency anemia. Microcytic anemia associated with increased red blood cell distribution width favors a diagnosis of iron deficiency anemia over that of anemia of chronic disease. The peripheral blood smear in iron deficiency anemia usually shows anisocytosis and poikilocytosis. Iron deficiency anemia may be associated with reactive thrombocytosis. In contrast, microcytic anemia associated with increased red blood cell count is characteristic of the thalassemia trait. Polychromasia, basophilic stippling, and target cells are absent in iron deficiency anemia but are characteristic features of the peripheral blood smear in thalassemia.

If the serum ferritin level is normal, the physician should determine if the microcytic anemia is preexisting or new. If the microcytosis is preexisting, a diagnosis of thalassemia should be considered. If the microcytosis is new, the differential diagnosis includes anemia of chronic disease and hereditary or acquired sideroblastic anemia. Anemia of chronic disease is usually normocytic, but may be microcytic in some systemic diseases such as temporal arteritis, rheumatoid arthritis, polymyalgia rheumatica, diabetes mellitus, connective tissue disease, chronic infection, Hodgkin's lymphoma, and renal cell carcinoma. The diagnosis is made on clinical grounds, and the microcytic anemia often is accompanied by systemic signs and symptoms.

Normocytic Anemia

The evaluation of normocytic anemia begins by identifying treatable causes such as nutritional anemias, anemia of renal insufficiency, bleeding, and hemolytic anemia. The initial investigation should include a fecal occult blood test and determination of serum ferritin, serum vitamin B_{12}, and serum folate levels. The diagnosis of anemia of renal insufficiency may be made on the basis of an elevated serum creatinine. Mild to moderate anemia may be seen when the serum creatinine is 1.5–3 mg/dL, while more severe anemia is found with more advanced renal disease. Anemia of renal insufficiency is associated with an unremarkable peripheral blood smear and a normal serum erythropoietin level.

If hemolysis is suspected, this diagnosis may be supported by a low haptoglobin level and increased lactate dehydrogenase (LDH), indirect bilirubin, and reticulocyte count. These tests are not specific and do not distinguish among the various causes of hemolytic anemia. The peripheral blood smear guides the evaluation of a suspected hemolytic anemia and is outlined in further detail below.

If a normocytic anemia is not linked to bleeding, nutrition, renal insufficiency, or hemolysis, the differential diagnosis includes a primary bone marrow disorder or normocytic anemia of chronic disease. The patient's history and peripheral blood smear may help to differentiate these two diagnoses, and hematology consultation should be considered. Other possible causes of normocytic anemia are alcohol abuse, drug effects, radiation therapy, chemical exposure, and recent trauma or surgery.

Macrocytic Anemia

The evaluation of macrocytic anemia begins by excluding alcohol or drug use associated with macrocytosis. Drugs associated with macrocytosis include hydroxyurea, methotrexate, trimethoprim, zidovudine, and 5-fluorouracil.

Vitamin B_{12} and folate deficiencies must be ruled out. In vitamin B_{12} deficiency, the serum vitamin B_{12} levels are usually low, but may be falsely low in elderly patients, in patients with low white blood cell counts, and in pregnant patients. The serum methylmalonic acid level is a more sensitive and highly specific test. A normal level makes the diagnosis of vitamin B_{12} deficiency very unlikely. In folate deficiency, serum folate levels are usually low, but may be affected by recent dietary changes. The serum homocysteine level is increased during folate deficiency and may be used instead to evaluate for folate deficiency.

If vitamin B_{12} deficiency is confirmed, intrinsic factor antibodies should be ordered. If they are present, a working diagnosis of pernicious anemia is made. If intrinsic factor antibodies are not present, the Schilling test can help differentiate pernicious anemia from primary intestinal malabsorptive disorders.

If vitamin deficiency, alcohol abuse, or drug exposure cannot be implicated as the cause of a macrocytic anemia, the process should be classified into mild (MCV 100–100 fL) or marked (MCV >110 fL) macrocytosis. Marked macrocytosis that is not due to nutritional deficiency, alcohol, or drug abuse usually is associated with a primary bone marrow disease such as myelodysplastic syndrome, aplastic anemia, or pure red cell aplasia. A bone marrow biopsy should be considered if the hematologic diagnosis affects management decisions. For a mild macrocytosis, the peripheral blood smear should be examined for evidence of an association with diseases such as liver disease or hypothyroidism. Bone marrow biopsy may be necessary to clarify the diagnosis.

Causes of Anemia

Microcytic Anemia

- Anemia of chronic disease
- Iron deficiency anemia
- Sideroblastic anemia
- Thalassemia

Normocytic Anemia

- Acute blood loss
- Anemia of chronic disease
- Autoimmune hemolytic anemias (warm-reactive anemias, cold-reactive anemias, drug-induced anemias)
- Chronic renal failure
- Endocrine deficiency states (hypothyroidism, adrenal insufficiency, pituitary deficiency, hypogonadism)
- Glucose-6-phosphate dehydrogenase deficiency
- Hemoglobinopathies (sickle cell disease and sickle hemoglobin C disease)
- Hereditary elliptocytosis
- Hereditary spherocytosis
- Hypersplenism
- Hyperthyroidism
- Liver disease
- Macrovascular disorders
- Marrow hypoplasia or aplasia
- Microangiopathic disorders (disseminated intravascular coagulopathy, hemolytic–uremic syndrome, thrombotic thrombocytopenic purpura)
- Myelopathies
- Myeloproliferative diseases
- Overhydration
- Paroxysmal nocturnal hemoglobinuria
- Pregnancy

- Pure red blood cell aplasia
- Pyruvate kinase deficiency
- Sideroblastic anemias

Macrocytic Anemia

- Alcohol abuse
- Aplastic anemia
- Clonal hematologic disorder
- Drug-induced
- Hemolytic anemia
- Large granular lymphocyte disorder
- Liver disease
- Myelodysplastic syndrome
- Nutritional
- Spurious

Key Historical Features

✓ Fever

✓ Fatigue

✓ Weakness

✓ Dyspnea

✓ Dizziness

✓ Apathy

✓ Cognitive impairment

✓ Worsening congestive heart failure

✓ Pruritis

✓ Dark urine

✓ Hematuria

✓ Back pain

Key Physical Findings

✓ Vital signs

✓ Evidence of conjunctival pallor

✓ Skin examination for jaundice or pallor

✓ Cardiac examination for tachycardia or flow murmur

✓ Lymphadenopathy

✓ Abdominal examination for hepatosplenomegaly

✓ Extremity examination for leg ulcers

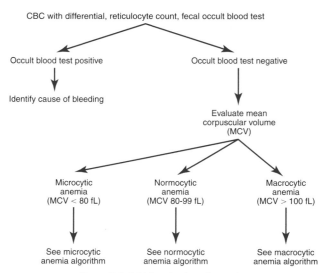

Figure 5-1. Initial evaluation of anemia.

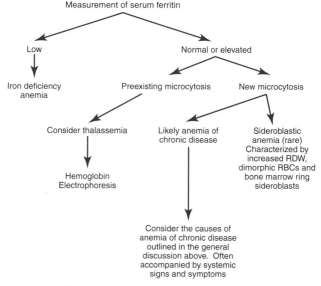

Figure 5-2. Evaluation of microcytic anemia.

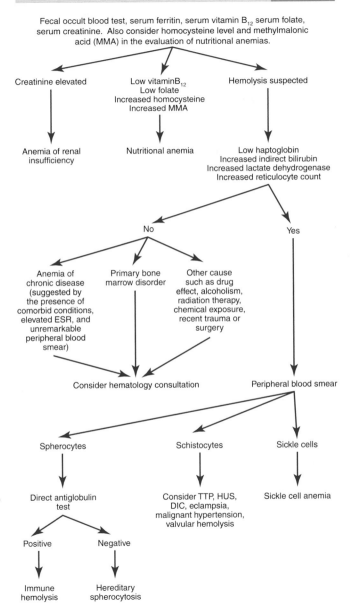

Figure 5-3. Evaluation of normocytic anemia.

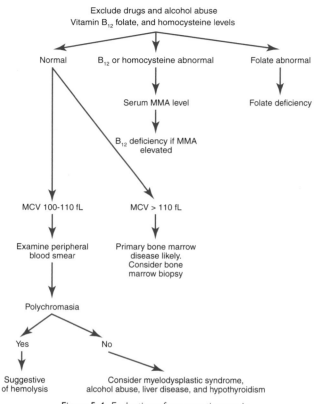

Figure 5-4. Evaluation of macrocytic anemia.

Further reading

Abramson SD, Abramson N. 'Common' uncommon anemias. American Family Physician 1999;59: 851–858.

Brill JR, Baumgardner DJ. Normocytic anemia. American Family Physician 2000;62: 2255–2263.

Dhaliwal G, Cornett PA, Tierney Jr. LM. Hemolytic anemia. American Family Physician 2004;69: 2599–2606.

Smith DL. Anemia in the elderly. American Family Physician 2000;62: 1565–1572.

Tefferi A, Hanson CA, Inwards DJ. How to interpret and pursue an abnormal complete blood cell count in adults. Mayo Clinic Proceedings 2005;80: 923–936.

Tefferi A. Anemia in adults: a contemporary approach to diagnosis. Mayo Clinic Proceedings 2003;78: 1274–1280.

6 ARTHRITIS AND ARTHRALGIA

General Discussion

Several different terms are often used to describe joint disorders resulting in joint pain. Arthralgia means joint pain. Arthritis implies the presence of an inflammatory component to the disorder. Arthropathy is a general term meaning joint disease but usually means that there is some degree of cartilage damage. Rheumatoid disease, infection, and crystal deposition are examples of conditions which produce an inflammatory response and a resultant cartilage loss. Osteoarthritis, or degenerative joint disease, occurs primarily as a result of cartilage breakdown, but often has a component of secondary inflammation. This chapter focuses on arthritis; however, some of the medications and conditions listed below may cause arthralgia without an inflammatory process.

Before attributing a patient's pain to arthritis, the physician must consider other potential causes of the pain. These potential diagnoses include intra-articular processes distinct from arthritis (impingement, neoplasm) as well as periarticular sources of pain (bursitis, tendonitis). Patients may also have referred pain from an adjacent site or a distant site as occurs with radiculopathy and spinal stenosis.

Medications Associated with Arthritis/Arthralgias

Acyclovir

Adalimumab

Amiodarone

Amphotericin

Atorvastatin

Beta blockers

Bacille Calmette–Guérin (BCG) vaccine

Carbamazepine

Chlorpromazine

Cyclosporine

Diuretics

Erythropoietin

Estrogens

Etanercept

Ethambutol

Fibrates

Fluoride

Granulocyte-colony stimulating factor (G-CSF)

Gold salts

Griseofulvin

Hydralazine

Infliximab

Interferons

Interleukin-2 and interleukin-6

Isoniazid

Letrozole

Levodopa

Lithium

Methimazole

Methyldopa

Minocycline

Nicardipine

Nicotinic acid

Para-aminosalicylic acid

Penicillin

Penicillamine

Phenytoin

Procainamide

Propylthiouracil

Pyrazinamide

Quinidine

Quinolones

Raloxifene

Reserpine

Simvastatin

Steroids (systemic)

Sulfasalazine

Tacrolimus

Tamoxifen

Terbinafine

Tetracycline

Ticlopidine

Vitamin A excess

Causes of Arthritis

Ankylosing spondylitis

Degenerative joint disease (osteoarthritis)

Giant cell arteritis

Gout

Hemochromatosis

Hemophilia

Infection

- Atypical mycobacteria
- Bacterial (*Staphylococcus aureus, Streptococcus, Salmonella, Neisseria gonorrhoeae, Haemophilus influenza, Escherichia coli, Pseudomonas*)
- Fungi (*Coccidioides immitis, Histoplasma capsulatum, Blastomyces dermatitides*)
- Gonorrhea
- HIV arthritis
- Lyme disease
- Tuberculosis
- Viral (HIV, hepatitis B, hepatitis C, parvovirus B19, rubella, Coxsackieviruses, alphaviruses, HTLV-1)

Immune reconstitution syndrome following highly active anti-retroviral therapy

Infectious endocarditis

Inflammatory bowel disease

Medications

Polymyalgia rheumatica

Pseudogout (calcium pyrophosphate dehydrate crystal deposition disease)

Psoriatic arthritis

Reactive arthritis (immunologic reaction to a prior infection)

Referred pain or pain from intra-articular disease other than arthritis

- Bursitis
- Impingement syndromes
- Neoplasm
- Spinal stenosis
- Radiculopathy
- Tendinitis

Rheumatoid arthritis

Scleroderma

Seronegative spondyloarthropathies

Sickle cell anemia

Still's disease

Systemic lupus erythematosus

Trauma

Whipple's disease

Key Historical Features

✓   Distribution/location of pain

✓   Quantification of pain

✓   Description of pain

✓   Radiation

✓   Duration and timing of symptoms

✓   Swelling

✓   Morning stiffness

✓   Degree of functional impairment

✓   Pain that wakes the patient

✓   Effect of treatment modalities

✓   Mechanic symptoms such as catching, locking, or joint instability

✓   Systemic symptoms such as fever, weight loss, night sweats, or fatigue

✓   Past medical history, especially previous trauma to the affected joint

✓   Past surgical history, especially surgery on the affected joint

✓   Medications

✓   Family history of arthritis

✓   Social history, including smoking, alcohol use, illicit drug use

✓   Occupational history, especially for jobs associated with repetitive trauma

✓   Review of systems for constitutional symptoms, urethritis, conjunctivitis, or skin lesions

Key Physical Findings

✓   Inspection

- •   Posture
- •   Body habitus
- •   Use of mobility aids
- •   Gait
- •   Leg length discrepancy

- • Scars from previous trauma or surgery
- • Swelling
- • Erythema
- • Muscle atrophy
- • Deformity of shape or alignment
- • Skin lesions

✓ Palpation

- • Warmth
- • Effusion
- • Tenderness to palpation over individual structures

✓ Range of motion

- • Active and passive range of motion testing
- • Presence of crepitus

✓ Muscle testing

✓ Ligament testing for laxity and joint instability

Suggested Work-Up

Radiographs of the affected joint	For most patients presenting with chronic, progressive joint pain, recent joint trauma, history of childhood joint problems, or night pain. Suggested radiographic views are outlined below.
CBC, rheumatoid factor (RF), antinuclear antibodies (ANA), ESR	Screening for any patient in whom rheumatoid and seronegative arthropathies are in the differential diagnosis
Serum uric acid level	For any patient with an inflammatory arthropathy in the absence of infection to evaluate for gouty arthritis
CBC and ESR	If septic arthritis is in the differential diagnosis
Joint aspiration and synovial fluid analysis	For any patient with suspected infection or suspected crystal-induced arthritis (see chapter on synovial fluid analysis)

Additional Work-Up

Technetium 99 m bone scan	If plain radiographs show a lesion suggestive of metastatic tumor, a total bone scan of the body can evaluate for metastatic tumor except multiple myeloma
MRI of the affected area, serum protein electrophoresis (SPEP), and urine protein electrophoresis (UPEP)	If multiple myeloma is suspected
CBC, ESR, uric acid, rheumatoid factor, urethral swab for Chlamydia, stool culture, synovial fluid gram stain, culture, and crystal analysis	If reactive arthritis is suspected

Suggested Radiographic Views

Anterior hip (groin)	AP pelvis
	Lateral view of affected hip
Posterior hip/buttock	AP pelvis (sacroiliac joints)
	AP/lateral lumbar spine
Knee	Standing AP both knees
	Lateral of affected knee
	Merchant view
Ankle	AP, lateral, and mortise views
Foot	Standing AP, lateral, and oblique views
Low back	AP/lateral lumbar spine
	Obliques (facet joints)

	Fergusson view (L5-S1 upshot)
Neck	AP/lateral C-spine
	Obliques (foraminal stenosis)
	Flexion/extension in rheumatoids
Shoulder	True AP of scapula
	Axillary lateral
Systemic arthritis	Views of primarily affected joints
	AP/lateral of hands and wrists

Further reading

Calabrese LH, Naides SJ. Viral arthritis. Infectious Disease Clinics of North America 2005; 19: 963–980.

Dearborn JT, Jergesen HE. The evaluation and initial management of arthritis. Primary Care: Clinics in Office Practice 1996;23: 215–240.

Harrington L, Schneider JI. Atraumatic joint and limb pain in the elderly. Emergency Medicine Clinics of North America 2006;24: 389–412.

Petersel DL, Sigal LH. Reactive arthritis. Infectious Disease Clinics of North America 2005; 19: 863–883.

Quiceno GA, Cush JJ. Iatrogenic rheumatic syndromes in the elderly. Clinics in Geriatric Medicine 2005;21: 577–588.

Raj JM, Sudhakar S, Sems, K, Carlson RW. Arthritis in the intensive care unit. Critical Care Clinics 2002;18: 767–780.

Rindfleisch JA, Muller D. Diagnosis and management of rheumatoid arthritis. American Family Physician 2005;72: 1037–1047.

General Discussion

In the United States, approximately 80% of ascites is caused by cirrhosis while nonhepatic causes account for the remaining 20%. In patients with liver disease, portal hypertension leads to ascites formation. Paracentesis should be performed on all patients with new-onset, clinically apparent ascites.

The incidence of ascitic fluid infection is 10–27% at the time of hospital admission. Patients with ascitic fluid infection may present with subtle symptoms, and early detection of infection with treatment at an early stage reduces morbidity and mortality. Diagnostic paracentesis should be repeated if a patient with ascites develops fever, abdominal pain, hypotension, abdominal tenderness, renal failure, encephalopathy, peripheral leukocytosis, or acidosis.

The serum-ascites albumin gradient (SAAG) is useful in determining the cause of ascites and guiding management. When the SAAG is equal to or greater than 1.1 g/dL, the patient has portal hypertension as the cause of ascites. The differential diagnosis includes cirrhosis, alcoholic hepatitis, hepatocellular carcinoma, massive liver metastases, fulminant hepatic failure, cardiac ascites, myxedema, Budd–Chiari syndrome, portal vein thrombosis, veno-occlusive disease of the liver, acute fatty liver of pregnancy, and mixed ascites.

When the SAAG is less than 1.1 g/dL, portal hypertension is not the cause of ascites. The differential diagnosis includes peritoneal carcinomatosis, tuberculous peritonitis, Chlamydia peritonitis, pancreatic ascites, biliary ascites, peritonitis from connective tissue disease such as lupus, bowel infarction, bowel perforation, and postoperative lymphatic leakage. Peritoneal carcinomatosis is the most common cause of ascites in patients with a low SAAG.

Ascitic fluid polymorphonuclear (PMN) leukocyte count is a more reliable indicator for infection than ascitic fluid white blood cell count. In calculating the PMN count, one PMN is subtracted from the absolute ascitic fluid PMN count for every 250 red blood cells. A corrected ascitic fluid PMN count greater than 250 cells/mm^3 should be treated as an ascitic fluid infection until proven otherwise.

Causes of Ascites

AIDS

Biliary tree leakage

Chemical burn to the peritoneum causing biliary or pancreatic ascites

Chlamydia (Fitz–Hugh–Curtis syndrome)

Coccidiomycosis

Congestive heart failure

Constrictive pericarditis

Endometriosis

Eosinophilic gastroenteritis

Familial Mediterranean fever

Glove starch peritonitis

Hepatic vein thrombosis

Hereditary angioedema

Histoplasmosis

Intrahepatic portal hypertension

Lymphoma

Meig's syndrome

Mesenteric lymphatic leakage

Mesothelioma

Metastatic cancer

Mixed ascites from two causes of fluid retention

Myxedema

Nephrogenic ascites in patients receiving hemodialysis

Nephrotic syndrome

Ovarian hyperstimulation syndrome

Pancreatic duct or pseudocyst leakage

Peritoneal carcinomatosis

Pneumatosis cystoids intestinalis

Portal vein thrombosis

Systemic lupus

Tuberculosis

Key Historical Features

✓ Presence of fever

✓ Presence of abdominal pain

✓ Past medical history

✓ Past surgical history

✓ Medications

✓ Family history of liver disease

✓ Risk factors for liver disease

- Blood transfusions
- Sexual practices
- Alcohol use
- Drug use
- Tattoos
- Acupuncture
- Body piercings
- Country of origin
✓ Tuberculosis exposures
✓ Review of systems with focus on potential for congestive heart failure or cancer

Key Physical Findings

✓ Vital signs

✓ Cardiac examination for signs suggestive of right heart failure such as abnormal jugular venous distension and systolic pulsation of the jugular veins or liver. Examination for signs of constrictive pericarditis such as pulsus paradoxicus or Kussmaul's sign

✓ Abdominal examination for shifting dullness to percussion, tympany, a fluid wave, hepatomegaly, or splenomegaly

✓ Back exam for venous distension

✓ Extremity examination for edema

✓ Evidence of chronic liver disease such as vascular spiders, splenomegaly, or distended abdominal collateral veins

✓ Evidence of malignancy such as an umbilical nodule or enlarged left supraclavicular lymph node

Suggested Work-Up

Serum albumin	Used to calculate the SAAG
Ascitic fluid albumin level	Used to calculate the SAAG
Ascitic fluid cell count	PMN count is usually more than 70% of the ascitic fluid WBC count in the setting of spontaneous bacterial peritonitis. Elevated WBC with lymphocytic predominance suggests tuberculous peritonitis or peritoneal carcinomatosis

Ascitic fluid total protein level	High ascitic fluid total protein level may suggest peritoneal carcinomatosis, tuberculous peritonitis, cardiac ascites, Budd-Chiari syndrome, myxedema, lymphatic rupture, intestinal perforation, biliary ascites, or pancreatic ascites
Ascitic fluid gram stain and culture	To evaluate for infection (aerobic and anaerobic)
Serum and ascitic fluid glucose	Used to evaluate for infection. Ascitic fluid glucose is lower than serum levels in the presence of infection
Serum and ascitic fluid LDH	Used to evaluate for infection. LDH levels may rise above that in the serum during infection
Ascitic fluid amylase	Amylase level in uncomplicated ascites is about 44% that in serum but rises significantly with pancreatitis and gut perforation

Additional Work-Up

Ascitic fluid triglycerides	Should be obtained if the ascitic fluid is opalescent or milky because chylous ascitic fluid has a triglyceride level of at least 200 mg/dL. Chylous ascites is caused by lymphatic rupture, usually due to cirrhosis or lymphoma
Ascitic fluid bilirubin	Should be tested if the ascitic fluid is dark brown. An ascitic fluid bilirubin level >6 mg/dL and greater than the serum level suggests biliary or upper gut perforation
Ascitic fluid cytology	If malignancy is a potential diagnosis. However, positive cytologic results are expected only in peritoneal carcinomatosis. Hepatocellular carcinoma, liver metastases, and lymphoma usually do not produce positive cytology results unless there are metastases to the peritoneum
Peritoneal biopsy by laparoscopy (sent for acid fast bacteria (AFB) stains and cultures)	If tuberculosis is suspected

Further reading

Cardenas A, Bataller R, Arroyo V. Mechanisms of ascites formation. Clinics in Liver Disease 2000;4: 447–465.

Midha NK, Stratton CW. Laboratory tests in critical care. Critical Care Clinics 1998; 14: 15–34.

Reynolds TB. Ascites. Clinics in Liver Disease 2000;4: 151–168.

Yu AS, Hu KQ. Management of ascites. Clinics in Liver Disease 2001;5: 541–568.

8 ATRIAL FIBRILLATION

General Discussion

Atrial fibrillation is the most common sustained arrhythmia treated by the physician. The incidence of atrial fibrillation increases with age and approximately doubles with each decade of life. The incidence of atrial fibrillation is further affected by the presence of both chronic medical illnesses and acute precipitating factors, which are outlined below. Myocardial infarction can be complicated by atrial fibrillation. However, patients presenting with atrial fibrillation without chest pain, anginal equivalent, or electrocardiogram (EKG) changes suggestive of ischemia are unlikely to have silent heart disease. The general consensus is that these patients do not need to be worked up for ischemia. In approximately 3% of patients with atrial fibrillation, no apparent cause is identified.

When atrial fibrillation is identified, the decision must be made whether the patient should be hospitalized. Indications for hospitalization include hemodynamic or cardiovascular instability, difficulty achieving rate control, or significant symptoms related to the arrhythmia. Hospitalization may also be indicated for patients who are candidates for early cardioversion.

Conditions Associated with Atrial Fibrillation

Cardiac Disease

- Atrial amyloidosis
- Cardiac arrhythmias
- Cardiac tumor
- Cardiomyopathy
- Congenital heart disease
- Coronary artery disease
- Left ventricular hypertrophy
- Myocarditis
- Pericarditis
- Rheumatic heart disease
- Valvular disease

Cerebrovascular accident

Diabetes mellitus

Exertion-induced

Hypertension

Increased sympathetic activity

- Anxiety
- Caffeine

- Drugs
- Hyperthyroidism
- Pheochromocytoma

Intoxicants

- Alcohol
- Amphetamines
- Carbon monoxide
- Cocaine
- Poison gas

Postoperative states

Pulmonary disease

- COPD
- Pulmonary embolism
- Pulmonary hypertension

Subarachnoid hemorrhage

Key Historical Features

✓ Precipitating factors for arrhythmia

✓ Symptoms associated with the arrhythmia

- Angina
- Change in exertional capacity
- Diaphoresis
- Dizziness
- Fatigue
- Palpitations
- Shortness of breath
- Syncope

✓ Past medical history

✓ Past surgical history, especially recent surgery

✓ Use of illicit substances

Key Physical Findings

✓ Vital signs for evidence of hemodynamic instability

✓ Cardiac examination

✓ Pulmonary examination

✓ Signs of atherosclerosis

- Arterial bruits

✓   Signs of heart failure

- Jugular venous distension

Suggested Work-Up

Electrocardiogram	To identify rhythm, signs of left ventricular hypertrophy, myocardial infarction, and pre-excitation
Chest X-ray	To evaluate the lung parenchyma and pulmonary vasculature
Echocardiogram	To identify valvular heart disease, left ventricular hypertrophy, atrial size, left ventricular size and function, peak right ventricular pressure, and pericardial disease. May identify left atrial thrombus
TSH	To evaluate for hyperthyroidism

Additional Work-Up

Exercise testing	To rule out coronary artery disease in patients suspected of having ischemia or who are at increased risk for coronary artery disease
Urinary metanephrines	If pheochromocytoma is suspected based upon the history and physical examination

Further reading

Jahangir A, Munger TM, Packer DL, et al. Atrial fibrillation. PJ.PR. Cardiac arrhythmias; mechanism, diagnosis, and management. Philadelphia: Lippincott Williams & Wilkins; 2001:457–499.

Kannel WB, Abbott RD, Savage DD, et al. Epidemiological features of chronic atrial fibrillation; the Framingham Study. New England Journal of Medicine 1982;306: 1018–1022.

Pelosi F, Morady F. Evaluation and management of atrial fibrillation. Medical Clinics of North America 2001;85: 225–244.

Podrid PJ. Atrial fibrillation in the elderly. Cardiology Clinics 1999;17: 173–188.

Ziv O, Coudhary G. Atrial fibrillation. Primary Care: Clinics in Office Practice 2005;32: 1083–1107.

General Discussion

Abnormal bleeding or bruising may cause significant anxiety for the patient and may be a sign of a serious inherited or acquired disorder. A history of bleeding following dental extraction, minor surgery, or childbirth suggests an underlying hemostatic disorder. Bleeding that is severe enough to require a blood transfusion merits particular attention. A family history of bleeding abnormalities suggests an inherited systemic disorder such as von Willebrand disease.

Bleeding from a platelet disorder typically is localized to superficial sites such as the skin or mucous membranes and usually is easily controlled. However, bleeding from hemostatic or plasma coagulation defects may occur hours or days after injury and is difficult to control with local measures. This type of bleeding often occurs into muscles, joints, or body cavities.

A thorough history is the most important step in establishing the presence of a hemostatic disorder and in guiding initial laboratory testing.

Medications Associated with Bleeding

Abciximab

Aspirin

Chemotherapeutic agents

Clopidogrel

Dalteparin

Enoxaparin

Eptifibatide

Heparin

Nonsteroidal anti-inflammatory drugs

Phenytoin

Quinine

Recombinant t-Pas (Activase and Retavase)

Ticlopidine

Tinzaparin

Tirofiban

Urokinase

Warfarin

Causes of Bleeding

Acquired factor VIII inhibitors

Acute leukemia

Adenocarcinoma

Alpha$_2$-antiplasmin deficiency

Aplastic anemia

Bernard-Soulier disease

Bone marrow failure

Chronic renal failure

Congenital factor deficiencies

Disseminated intravascular coagulation

Drug-related thrombocytopenia

Fat embolism

Glanzmann's disease

Hemolysis, Elevated Liver Enzymes, Low Platelet Count (HELLP) syndrome

Hemolytic uremic syndrome

Heparin-induced thrombocytopenia

HIV infection

Idiopathic thrombocytopenic purpura

Liver disease

Lyme disease

Lymphoma

Medications

Postprostatectomy hemorrhage

Post-transfusion purpura syndrome

Rat poison ingestion (superwarfarins)

Scott's syndrome

Storage pool disease

Systemic lupus erythematosus

Thrombotic thrombocytopenic purpura

Viral infections

Vitamin K deficiency

Von Willebrand disease

Key Historical Features

✓ Duration of the symptoms

✓ Mucous membrane bleeding (menorrhagia, epistaxis, gum bleeding)

✓ Bleeding into soft tissues such as muscles and joints

✓   Excessive bleeding during surgical procedures, fractures, or serious injuries

✓   Past medical history

✓   Past surgical history

✓   Medications

✓   Family history of bleeding

Key Physical Findings

✓   Epistaxis or bleeding from the gums

✓   Evaluation of the skin for purpura, ecchymoses, or hematomas

✓   Evidence of bleeding into muscles or joints

✓   Hepatomegaly

✓   Splenomegaly

Suggested Work-Up

CBC	To evaluate for aplastic anemia
Platelet count	To evaluate for thrombocytopenia
Peripheral blood smear	To evaluate the cell lines
Bleeding time	To evaluate platelet function
Prothrombin time	To evaluate plasma coagulation function
Activated partial thromboplastin time	To evaluate plasma coagulation function

Additional Work-Up

Thrombin time	Used when both the prothrombin time (PT) and activated partial thromboplastin time (PTT) are prolonged to test for fibrinogen conversion to fibrin
Factor VIII, von Willebrand factor antigen, von Willebrand factor activity (ristocetin cofactor assay), and template bleeding time	If von Willebrand disease is suspected

Prothrombin time, activated partial thromboplastin time, thrombin time, platelet count, factor VIII assay, factor V assay, fibrinogen, and D-dimer

If disseminated intravascular coagulation is suspected

Further reading

Ewenstein BM. The pathophysiology of bleeding disorders presenting as abnormal uterine bleeding. American Journal of Obstetrics and Gynecology 1996;175: 770–777.

Handin RI. Bleeding and thrombosis. In: Isselbacher KJ, Braunwald E, Wilson JD, eds. Harrison's Textbook of internal medicine, 13th ed. New York: McGraw-Hill; 1994:317–322.

Lusher JM. Screening and diagnosis of coagulation disorders. American Journal of Obstetrics and Gynecology 1996;175: 778–783.

McKenna R. Abnormal coagulation in the postoperative period contributing to excessive bleeding. Medical Clinics of North America 2001;85: 1277–1310.

10 CEREBROSPINAL FLUID EVALUATION

General Discussion

The central nervous system (CNS) is susceptible to bacterial, viral, and fungal infections, as well as to prion diseases and numerous local and systemic diseases. Examination of the cerebrospinal fluid (CSF) is crucial in helping to diagnose infections and other diseases. Although not definitive, certain CSF findings are suggestive of bacterial, viral, fungal, or tuberculous meningitis. These findings are outlined in Table 10.1 below.

These typical findings, in combination with specific antigen, antibody, and polymerase chain reaction tests may help to reveal the origin of a CNS infection or disease. The tests that are ordered on the CSF should be guided by the suspected underlying cause of the patient's illness. Recommended CSF studies based upon specific disorders are outlined in Table 10.2 below.

In patients who have bacterial meningitis and who receive antibiotics before lumbar puncture is performed, CSF abnormalities such as elevated white blood cell (WBC) count, elevated protein concentration, and depressed glucose may persist for one to three days, while results of Gram stain and culture of the CSF can become negative within hours after the antibiotics are administered. A mononuclear pleocytosis is usually present in patients who have viral meningitis, but it can be preceded by a transient predominance of polymorphonucleocytes for 8 to 48 hours. Elevated levels of CSF adenosine deaminase have a high sensitivity and specificity for tuberculous meningitis in adults.

For bacterial meningitis, CSF Gram stain and culture are the diagnostic tests of choice. Blood culture may also help identify the causative organism.

CSF Parameter	Bacterial Meningitis	Viral Meningitis	Fungal Meningitis	Tuberculous Meningitis
Opening pressure (mm H_2O)	>180	Often normal	Variable	>180
WBC count (cells/mm³)	1000–10 000 Range: <100–20 000	<300 Range: 100–1000	20–500 Variable, dependent upon fungus	50–500 Range: <50–4000
Neutrophils (%)	>80	<20	Usually <50	20
Protein (mg/dL)	100–500	Often normal	Elevated	150–200
Glucose (mg/dL)	<40	>40	Usually <40	<40
Gram stain (% positive)	60–90	Negative	Negative	37–87 (AFB smear)
Culture (% positive)	70–85	50	25–50	52–83

Table 10-1. Typical CSF Findings in Bacterial Meningitis

Domain	Disorder	Useful CSF Studies	Expected Results	Comments
Cerebral Dysfunction				
Infectious	Meningitis (purulent)	pr, gl, cell cts, gs, cx, op	↑ pr, ↓ gl, ↑ CSF PMNs, + gs and cx, + bacterial ags, ↑ op	+ cryptococcal ag and india ink in cryptococcal meningitis
			↑ LA	Mononuclear cells possible in partially rx'd bacterial meningitis
	Meningitis (aseptic)	pr, gl, cell cts	↑ pr, nl gl, ↑ CSF WBC (10 to 1000 mononuc cells/mm³)	PMNs possible in early aseptic meningitis
	Encephalitis	pr, gl, cell cts, gs, cx	mildly ↑ pr (50 to 100 mg/dL), nl gl, ↑ CSF WBC 50 to 100/mm³ (mononuc)	Herpes simplex encephalitis
			↑ RBC/xanthochromia, + CSF PCR	
	HIV encephalopathy	pr, gl, cell cts	mildly ↑ pr, nl gl, nl or few WBC	
	Neurosyphilis (acute)	VDRL, pr, gl	↑ pr (>45 mg/dL), ↑ WBC (5 to 500 mononuc/mm³), + VDRL	CSF parameters may be normal
	Neuroborreliosis	pr, gl, cell cts, OCB, abs	↑ pr (~100 mg/dL), nl or ↓ gl, ↑ WBC (~100 mononuc/mm³), + OCB, + Lyme abs	CSF normalizes in stage III
	Tuberculous meningitis	pr, gl, cell cts, op, acid-fast stain, cx	↑ pr (100 to 200 mg/dL), ↓ gl (<45 mg/dL), ↑ WBC (25 to 100 mononuc/mm³), ↑ op	May be spinal block; stain and culture require large amts. of CSF
	Abscess	Not recommended		May be dangerous to perform LP in the face of abscess; risk of herniation or ventricular rupture
	Creutzfeldt-Jakob	pr, gl, cell cts	Normal	14-3-3 protein in CSF (not readily available)

	Progressive multifocal leukoencephalopathy	JC virus PCR	+ JC virus PCR	CSF o/w normal
	Cysticercosis	pr, gl, cell cts, op	↑ pr, ↓ gl, ↑ WBC (mixed w/eosinophilia), ↑ op	CSF eosinophils constitute 20–75%
Cerebrovascular	Stroke	pr, cell cts	mildly ↑ pr and WBC	Not routinely performed; ↑ LDH, AST and CK-BB in cortical CVA
	Subarachnoid hemorrhage	pr, gl, cell cts, color	↑↑ pr, ↓ gl, ↑↑ RBC, ↑ WBC, xanth	pr can be normal or significantly ↑, gl can be normal or slightly ↓
	Venous thrombosis	cell cts, op	↑ RBC, ↑ op	WBC may be ↑ if 2° to septic thrombosis
	Anoxic brain			Not routinely performed; CK-BB, NSE, MBP may be useful
Dementia	Alzheimer's disease	pr, gl, cell cts	normal parameters	Abnormal CSF helps r/o AD
Degenerative	Huntington's disease	pr, gl, cell cts	normal	Abnormal CSF helps r/o Huntington's disease
	Wilson's disease	pr, gl, cell cts	normal	Abnormal CSF helps r/o Wilson's disease
Neoplastic	Meningeal carcinomatosis	pr, gl, cell cts, cyt, op	↑ pr (24 to 1200 mg/dL), ↓ gl, ↑ WBC (PMN), + cyt, mildly ↑ op	Large volumes of CSF and multiple LP's increase cytology yield
	Craniopharyngioma	cell cts	↑ WBC (mononuc)	A cause of chronic chemical meningitis
Metabolic	Hepatic encephalopathy	pr, color	↑ pr possible xanth	Not routinely performed; op may be ↑; CSF glutamine ↑
	Uremic encephalopathy	pr, cell cts, urea	mildly ↑ pr and WBC, ↑ urea,	Not routinely performed
	Myxedema coma	pr	↑ pr (100 to 300 mg/dL)	

Continued

Table 10-2. Selected Disorders and Associated CSF Studies

Domain	Disorder	Useful CSF Studies	Expected Results	Comments
Demyelinating	Mitochondrial encephalopathies	pyruvate, lactate	↑ pyruvate, lactate	MELAS
	Multiple sclerosis	pr, gl, cell cts, OCB, MBP, IgG index	↑ pr, mildly ↑ WBC, nl gl, + OCB, + MBP; ↑ IgG index	Abnormal CSF in 90% of cases; pr and cell cts nl in 2/3
	Acute disseminated encephalomyelitis	pr, gl cell cts, OCB	mildly ↑ pr and WBC, nl gl, + OCB	OCBs may disappear after resolution
Autoimmune	Sarcoid	pr, gl, cell cts	↑ pr (50 to 200 mg/dL), mildly ↓ gl (30 to 40 mg/dL), ↑ WBC (10 to 100 mononuc/mm³)	ACE ↑ in 50%, but not specific
	Behçet's disease	pr, cell cts	↑ pr, ↑ WBC (mixed response) 10 to 200 cell/mm³	CSF results quite varied
	Angiitis	pr, gl, cell cts, op	↑ pr, ↓ gl, ↑ WBC (mononuc), ↑ op	Abnormal CSF in 80–90%
Other disorders	Normal pressure hydrocephalus	Diagnostic high volume LP, op	Gait and mental status improvement after LP, nl op	High volume LP (40–50 cc of CSF)
	Pseudotumor cerebri	pr, cell cts, op	↓ pr, nl cell cts, ↑ op (250 to 600 mm H₂O)	CSF removal may be therapeutic in some cases
	Migraine	See comments		Little available data. May have ↑ pr and cell cts in severe complicated migraine
	Generalized seizure	pr, cell cts	nl ↑ pr, mild ↑ WBC	Postictal
	Reye's syndrome	pr, gl, cell cts, op	pr and gl nl, < 10 cell/mm³; ↑ op	
Cranial Nerve Dysfunction				
	Miller-Fisher variant of GBS	See GBS	See GBS/comments	Pr more commonly nl than in GBS

Optic neuritis	pr, cell cts, OCB	Mild ↑ pr (45 to 60 mg/dL), 50% with mild ↑ WBC (mononuc), + OCB	+ OCB increase risk o MS
Lyme disease	cell cts	Mild ↑ WBC (mononuc)	
Bell's palsy	pr, gl, cell cts	nl CSF	Abnormal CSF helps r/o Bell's palsy
Trigeminal neuralgia			Not routinely performed; may have ↑ substance P and ↓ monoamines
Kearns–Sayre syndrome	pr	↑ pr (70 to 400 mg/dL)	
Motor Dysfunction			
CNS			
Parkinson's disease			Not routinely performed. Abnormal CSF helps r/o Parkinson's disease
Huntington's disease	See above		Abnormal CSF helps r/o Huntington's disease
Wilson's disease	See above		Abnormal CSF helps r/o Wilson's disease
Neurosyphilis (paretic)	VDRL, pr, cell cts	++VDRL, pr: 50 to 100 mg/dL, cell cts: 25 to 75 leukocytes/mm^3	CSF abnormalities increase with duration of disease
HTLV-I	pr, gl, IgG, OCB	mild ↑ pr; nl gl; ↑ IgG, + OCB	Serum + HTLV-I ag
Poliomyelitis	pr, gl, cell cts	mild ↑ pr (50 to 200 mg/dL), nl gl, mild ↑ CSF WBC (mononuc)	CSF WBC ↓ with time
Spinal cord tumor	pr, gl, cell cts, cytology	may be ↑↑ pr; nl gl, ↑ WBC (mononuc), + cyt	Froin's syndrome (spinal cord block) may sig ↑

Table 10-2. Selected Disorders and Associated CSF Studies

Continued

Domain	Disorder	Useful CSF Studies	Expected Results	Comments
	Tetanus	pr; gl; cell cts	↑ pr (90 to 150 mg/dL), nl gl, nl cell cts	Care must be taken not to induce tetany. Normal cell cts differentiate from meningitis
	Stiffman's syndrome	pr; cell cts, IgG, OCB	nl pr; nl cell cts, ↑ IgG, ? + OCB	
Motor Neuron	ALS	pr; cell cts	mild ↑ pr and cell cts	Nondiagnostic
	GBS	pr; cell cts	↑ pr; nl cell cts	Pr peaks between 1 and 3 wks. Cell cts >5 should prompt search for another cause
Nerve	Brachial plexopathy	pr; cell cts	mild ↑ pr (50 to 60 mg/dL), nl cell cts	
	Chronic inflammatory demyelinating polyradiculopathy (CIDP)	pr; gl; cell cts	↑ pr (100 to 200 mg/dL), nl gl, mild ↑ WBC (5 to 50 cell/mm³)	Similar to GBS; pr elevation correlates with severity; + WBC in 10%
	Inherited neuropathy	pr; gl; cell cts	mod ↑ pr (50 to 200 mg/dL), nl cell cts	
Muscle	Myopathy or myositis			Not routinely performed
Cerebellar Dysfunction				
Cerebellitis		pr; gl; cell cts	mildly ↑ pr; nl gl; cell cts usually <100/mm² (mononuc)	Usually secondary to varicella-zoster
	Paraneoplastic cerebellar disease	pr; cell cts, abs	mild ↑ pr; mild ↑ WBC (8 to 20 cells/mm³) + anti-Yo or anti-Hu ab	Anti-Yo in ovarian, uterine, or breast CA. Anti-Hu seen in lung CA
Sensory Dysfunction				
Neuropathy	Diabetic	pr; gl; cell cts	↑ pr (50 to 400 mg/dL), nl cell cts. ↑ gl (secondary diabetes)	
	CIDP	See above		

Inherited neuropathies		See above	
Neurosyphilis (tabes dorsalis)	VDRL, pr, gl, cell cts	3/4 w/+ VDRL, CSF freq o/w WNL	CSF may resemble paretic form, but parameters improve w/progression

abs, Antibodies; ACE, angiotensin-converting enzyme; AD, Alzheimer's dementia; ag, antigen; AST, aspartate aminotransferase; bact, bacteria; CA, cancer; cell cts, cell counts; cerebrovasc, cerebrovascular; CK-BB, creatinine kinase BB isoenzyme; CSF, cerebrospinal fluid; CVA, cerebrovascular accident (stroke); cyt, cytology; degen, degenerative; GBS, Guillain-Barré syndrome; gl, glucose; gs, Gram stain; LA, lactic acid; LDH, lactate dehydrogenase; MBP, myelin basic protein; mononuc, mononuclear cells; nl, normal; NPH, normal pressure hydrocephalus; NSE, neuron-specific-enolase; OCB, oligoclonal bands; OP, opening; o/w, otherwise; pr, protein; r/o, rule out; rx'd, treated; sig, significantly; VDRL, venereal disease research laboratory test; wks, weeks; WNL, within normal limits; xanth, xanthochromia.

Table 10-2. Selected Disorders and Associated CSF Studies

CSF viral culture is able to detect 14 to 24% of cases of viral meningitis. Tuberculous and fungal meningitis may be difficult to diagnose by routine CSF smear or culture. CSF culture is positive in 52 to 83% of cases of tuberculous meningitis.

Cerebrospinal fluid cell counts with differentials should be performed on every specimen. Typically, the CSF contains no red blood cells (RBC)/µL and 0 to 1 WBC/µL. A traumatic lumbar puncture causes elevations of RBCs and WBCs, but these elevations are differentiated from subarachnoid hemorrhage because in a traumatic lumbar puncture the elevations are high in the first tube but clear in the later tubes. In subarachnoid hemorrhage, the elevations persist in each test tube. To determine whether an elevated CSF WBC is due to blood from a traumatic tap or other causes, an expected ratio may be used. If the elevated WBC is due to blood in the CSF, 1 WBC/µL for every 700 RBC/µL is found. If the WBC exceeds this ratio, its origin must be accounted for from other etiologies such as infection or inflammation.

The CSF glucose concentration is normally 60% of the plasma glucose concentration. It is important to obtain a serum glucose level at the time of the CSF sample. An elevated CSF glucose level results from an elevated plasma glucose level. A decreased CSF glucose concentration may be due to hypoglycemia, bacterial meningitis, fungal meningitis, certain viral meningitides, subarachnoid hemorrhage, carcinomatosis meningitis, chemical meningitis, and parasitic meningitis.

Elevation in CSF protein is a nonspecific but sensitive indicator of CNS disease. A CSF protein concentration greater than 500 mg/dL is an infrequent finding, but can occur with bacterial meningitis, subarachnoid hemorrhage, or spinal–subarachnoid block. When a significant amount of blood is present in the CSF, the total protein concentration can be corrected by reducing the protein by 1 mg/dL for every 1000 RBCs in the CSF. Protein concentrations of 100 mg/dL or greater have sensitivity and specificity for bacterial meningitis of 82 and 98%, respectively. If the concentration is 200 mg/dL, the sensitivity is 86% and the specificity is 100%.

The finding of oligoclonal bands in the CSF implies that a single clonal population of plasma cells is responsible for each band seen on gel electrophoresis. More than one oligoclonal band rarely occurs in normal CSF. A serum sample should be obtained simultaneously with a CSF sample to determine whether oligoclonal bands are unique to the CSF. Oligoclonal bands are present in 83 to 94% of patients with multiple sclerosis, and are also present in disorders such as subacute sclerosing panencephalitis, CNS lupus, neurosarcoidosis, cysticercosis, Behçet's syndrome, Guillain-Barré syndrome, some brain tumors, and viral, fungal, and bacterial infections.

Further reading

Coyle PK. Overview of acute and chronic meningitis. Neurologic Clinics 1999;17:691–710.
Goetz C. Textbook of clinical neurology, 2nd ed. Philadelphia: Saunders; 2003:511–524.

Huhn GD, Sejvar JJ, Montgomery SP, Dworkin MS. West nile virus in the United States: an update on an emerging infectious disease. American Family Physician 2003;68: 653–660.

Re VL, Gluckman SJ. Eosinophilic meningitis. The American Journal of Medicine 2003; 114: 217–223.

Teunissen CE, Dijkstra C, Polman C. Biologic markers in CSF and blood for axonal degeneration in multiple sclerosis. The Lancet Neurology 2005;4: 32–41.

Thomson RB, Bertram H. Laboratory diagnosis of central nervous system infections. Infectious Disease Clinics of North America 2001;15: 1047–1071.

Zunt JR, Marra CM. Cerebrospinal fluid testing for the diagnosis of central nervous system infection. Neurologic Clinics 1999;17: 675–689.

General Discussion

Chest pain is a very common complaint of patients presenting to the emergency room as well as to outpatient clinics. More than 50% of those patients presenting to the emergency department with chest pain have acute coronary syndrome (ACS), pulmonary embolism or heart failure. However, most patients presenting to outpatient departments have diseases such as stable angina, musculoskeletal disorders, gastrointestinal disease, pulmonary disease or psychiatric disorders.

The differential diagnosis of chest pain is broad and ranges from benign to potentially life-threatening. Fortunately, most cases of chest pain actually represent a much smaller list of disease processes. The history (especially risk factors for coronary artery disease), physical examination, and selected testing such as the electrocardiogram and chest X-ray can help narrow the differential diagnosis and focus further testing.

Medications Associated with Chest Pain

Azathioprine (pancreatitis)

Corticosteroids (pancreatitis)

Cyclosporine (pancreatitis)

Furosemide (pancreatitis)

NSAIDs (peptic ulcer disease)

Oral contraceptives (pancreatitis, pulmonary embolism)

Sulfonamides (pancreatitis)

Tacrolimus (pancreatitis)

Tetracycline (pancreatitis)

Thiazides (pancreatitis)

Valproic acid (pancreatitis)

Causes of Chest Pain

Breast pain

- Abscess
- Breast cancer
- Breast cyst
- Cyclic breast pain
- Mastitis

Cardiac causes

- Acute coronary syndrome (myocardial infarction, unstable angina)

- Aortic stenosis
- Coronary artery dissection
- Coronary artery spasm
- Heart failure
- Myocarditis
- Pericarditis
- Stable angina
- Thoracic aortic dissection (TAD)

Gastrointestinal causes

- Biliary disease
- Esophageal cancer
- Esophageal spasm
- Gastric cancer
- Gastroesophageal reflux disease
- Pancreatic cancer
- Pancreatitis
- Peptic ulcer disease

Musculoskeletal causes

- Contusion
- Costochondritis
- Disc disease (cervical or thoracic)
- Fibromyalgia
- Osteoarthritis
- Rib fracture
- Thoracic outlet syndrome
- Tietze's syndrome

Psychiatric causes

- Depression
- Factitious disorder
- Panic disorder
- Somatization

Pulmonary causes

- Bronchitis
- Lung cancer
- Pleuritis
- Pneumonia
- Pneumothorax
- Pulmonary embolism (PE)

Other causes

- Familial Mediterranean Fever
- Herpes zoster
- Mediastinal tumors

Key Historical Features

✓ Type of pain (pleuritic versus nonpleuritic; crushing pain versus sharp versus burning)

✓ Severity of pain

✓ Duration and onset of pain

✓ Location of pain

✓ Prior episodes of chest pain

✓ Exacerbating factors, especially exercise

✓ Relieving factors, especially rest or nitroglycerin

✓ Worsening of pain with certain movements

✓ Radiation of pain

✓ Relation of pain to meals

✓ History of trauma

✓ Fever

✓ Associated symptoms, especially potentially cardiac symptoms

- Syncope
- Dizziness
- Weakness
- Palpitations

✓ Medical History

- Risk factors for coronary artery disease: diabetes, hyperlipidemia, hypertension, prior history of coronary artery disease (CAD), family history of CAD, smoking history
- Review risk factors for PE: use of oral contraceptives, hormone replacement therapy, hypercoagulable state (malignancies, thrombophilias, pregnancy, recent surgery), recent travel, immobilization
- Review risk factors for TAD: hypertension, Marfan's syndrome, cocaine use

✓ Obstetric/Gynecologic History

- Evaluate possibility of pregnancy, which will affect the work-up and treatment

✓   Past Surgical History

✓   Medications

✓   Social history (smoking, alcohol use, drug use)

✓   Family history

✓   Review of systems

- Cardiac (see above)
- Gastrointestinal
  - Nausea and vomiting
  - Rectal bleeding
  - Abdominal pain
- Pulmonary
  - Cough may be a sign of pneumonia, lung cancer, heart failure or bronchitis
  - Hemoptysis may be a sign of pneumonia, lung cancer, pulmonary embolism, or heart failure
  - Dyspnea may be a sign of ACS, heart failure, pneumonia, pulmonary embolism, pneumothorax
- Neurologic
  - Evaluate for weakness or numbness due to a stroke which can be caused by TAD
- Psychiatric
  - Evaluate history of depression or anxiety. However, do not presume that symptoms are due to psychiatric illness

Physical Findings

✓   Vital signs, including pulse oximetry

✓   General assessment of well-being

✓   Cardiovascular examination for rhythm, rate, murmurs, heart sounds, apical impulse, peripheral pulses, and jugular venous distension

✓   Pulmonary examination for the presence of abnormal lung sounds, egophony, or dullness to percussion

✓   Abdominal examination for tenderness, organomegaly, or masses

✓   Rectal examination to evaluate for bleeding

✓   Neurologic examination for evidence of a stroke

✓   Skin examination for evidence of herpes zoster

✓ Musculoskeletal examination for evidence of chest wall, neck, or shoulder tenderness

✓ Extremity examination for evidence of deep vein thrombosis

Suggested Work-Up

In some patients, an adequate history and physical may be enough to determine that a patient has a non-threatening cause of chest pain. However, most patients will require at least an EKG, a chest X-ray and selected laboratory tests

Electrocardiogram	To evaluate for evidence of ischemia, pericarditis, pulmonary embolism, arrhythmias, or heart failure
Chest X-ray	To evaluate for pulmonary disease, heart failure, or thoracic aortic dissection
Serum markers of myocardial damage	To evaluate for acute coronary syndrome
Creatine kinase	
Creatine kinase-MB	
Troponin I	

Additional Work-Up

Complete blood count	To evaluate for infection or anemia
Amylase and/or lipase	If pancreatitis is suspected
AST, ALT, bilirubin	If liver or biliary disease is suspected
Abdominal ultrasound	If liver or biliary disease is suspected
Upper endoscopy	If peptic ulcer or gastric cancer is suspected
Mammogram	If a breast mass is palpated or the patient is due for breast cancer screening
CT scan of chest	If PE, TAD or lung cancer is suspected

D-dimer	When used in conjunction with scoring systems, a normal D-dimer along with a low pretest probability of a deep vein thrombosis or PE can be used to safely withhold further evaluation such as lower extremity compression ultrasound, ventilation-perfusion scanning, or CT angiogram
Ventilation perfusion scan or CT angiogram	If PE is suspected
Cardiac stress testing	If coronary artery disease is suspected
CT scan of abdomen	If an intra-abdominal malignancy, abscess or other process is suspected
Arterial blood gas	If the patient is hypoxic or has evidence of significant pulmonary disease
Blood cultures	If an infectious process is suspected
Sputum cultures	If pneumonia is suspected
Echocardiography	If heart failure, pericarditis, valvular disease, or other cardiac processes are suspected
Rib series (X-ray)	May be considered if rib fracture is suspected
Brain natriuretic peptide	If heart failure is suspected
Venous compression ultrasonography	To evaluate for a deep venous thrombosis in a patient who may have a PE

Further reading

Boie ET. Initial evaluation of chest pain. Emergency Medicine Clinics of North America 2005;23(4): 937–957.

Butler KH, Swencki SA. Chest pain: a clinical assessment. Radiologic Clinics of North America 2006;44(2): 165–179.

Cayley WE. Diagnosing the cause of chest pain. American Family Physician 2005;72(10): 2012–2021.

Douglas PS and Ginsburg GS. The evaluation of chest pain in women. New England Journal of Medicine 1996; 334(20):1311–1315.

Goldman L. Cecil Textbook of Medicine, 2nd ed. W.B. Saunders Company; 2004.

Pilote L, Dasgupta K, Guru V, et al. A comprehensive view of sex-specific issues related to cardiovascular disease. CMAJ 2007;176(6 suppl): S1–S44.

General Discussion

The cough reflex is complex, but cough generally results from irritant stimulation of one or more receptors in the respiratory system. Estimating the duration of cough is the first step in narrowing the list of possible diagnoses. Cough may be classified as acute (less than 3 weeks), subacute (3–8 weeks), or chronic (more than 8 weeks). If the cough is productive of blood, the patient should be evaluated according to guidelines for hemoptysis.

In non-smokers who do not take an ACE inhibitor and whose chest X-ray is normal, the most likely causes of chronic cough are asthma, postnasal drip, or gastroesophageal reflux disease (GERD). Other common causes in immunocompetent patients include chronic bronchitis due to cigarette smoking or other irritants, bronchiectasis, and eosinophilic bronchitis. The physician should assess the likelihood of the most common causes by means of trials of empirical therapy and trials involving the avoidance of irritants and drugs, along with focused laboratory testing such as chest radiography or methacholine challenge.

A normal chest radiograph in an immunocompetent patient makes postnasal drip syndrome, asthma, GERD, chronic bronchitis, and eosinophilic bronchitis more likely and bronchogenic carcinoma, tuberculosis, bronchiectasis, and sarcoidosis unlikely. If the chest radiograph is abnormal, the patient should be evaluated on the basis of the diseases suggested by the radiographic findings.

Postnasal drip syndrome is the most common cause of chronic cough and no diagnostic test exists, so the patient should be evaluated for this condition first. Next, asthma may be considered as a cause of chronic cough. A methacholine challenge should be considered since its negative predictive value is 100%. For the consideration of GERD, 24-hour monitoring of the esophagus is not routinely recommended because it is inconvenient for patients, is not widely available, and lacks sensitivity and specificity.

Although most chronic smokers have a cough, it should not be assumed that the cough is due to the smoking unless smoking ceases and the cough resolves. It is also important to recognize that multiple conditions often simultaneously contribute to cough. The definitive diagnosis of the cause of chronic cough is established on the basis of an observation of which specific therapy eliminates the cough. A chronic cough may be due to more than one condition 18 to 93% of the time, so therapy that is partially successful should not be stopped but should instead be sequentially supplemented.

If the patient has a history of smoking, is exposed to environmental irritants, or is currently being treated with an ACE inhibitor, the patient should be instructed to eliminate the irritant or discontinue the medication for 4 weeks. If the cough improves or resolves, the cough is partially or entirely due to chronic bronchitis or to the ACE inhibitor.

Eosinophilic bronchitis can be distinguished from asthma by the lack of bronchial hyperresponsiveness or variable airflow obstruction. Eosinophilic bronchitis should be considered in patients with negative methacholine challenge tests. It can be ruled out as a cause of chronic cough if eosinophils make up less than 3% of the nonsquamous cells in a sample of induced sputum.

Tuberculosis (TB) should be considered early in the evaluation of patients with chronic cough when the likelihood of tuberculosis is high. This includes areas where the prevalence of TB is high and in populations at high risk of TB such as HIV-infected persons. TB should also be considered in patients with chronic cough who have sputum production, hemoptysis, fever, or weight loss.

Causes of Chronic Cough

Aberrant innominate artery

ACE-inhibitor use

Asthma

Bronchiectasis

Bronchiolitis

Bronchogenic carcinomatosis

Chronic aspiration

Chronic bronchitis due to smoking or other irritants

Eosinophilic bronchitis

GERD

Interstitial lung disease

Irritable larynx

Left ventricular failure

Lymphoma

Metastatic carcinoma

Persistent pneumonia

Postinfectious cough

Postnasal drip (includes chronic sinusitis, allergic rhinitis, vasomotor rhinitis, and nonallergic rhinitis)

Pulmonary abscess

Psychogenic cough

Sarcoidosis

Tracheitis

Tuberculosis

Key Historical Features

✓ Fever

✓ Symptoms of asthma

✓ Heartburn or regurgitation

✓ Symptoms of postnasal drip (throat clearing, nasal discharge, excessive phlegm production)

✓ Exacerbating factors

✓ Diurnal variation

✓ Hemoptysis

✓ Purulent sputum

✓ Night sweats

✓ Weight loss

✓ Past medical history

✓ Medications, especially ACE inhibitor

✓ Tobacco use

✓ Environmental exposures

✓ HIV risk factors

Key Physical Findings

✓ Vital signs

✓ Head and neck examination for lymphadenopathy, nasal discharge, sinus tenderness, a cobblestone appearance of the oropharynx, mucus in the oropharynx

✓ Cardiac examination for evidence of left ventricular failure

✓ Pulmonary examination for any abnormal breath sounds

✓ Extremity examination for cyanosis or clubbing

Suggested Work-Up

Chest X-ray	Optional in the initial evaluation of younger nonsmokers with suspected postnasal drip syndrome or sinusitis

Additional Work-Up

Methacholine challenge	Useful in ruling out asthma as it has a negative predictive value of 100% in the context of cough

Bronchoscopy	Should be considered when the cause of cough remains unclear after an initial evaluation
Evaluation of induced sputum	May be helpful in diagnosing nonasthmatic eosinophilic bronchitis
High-resolution computerized tomography of the chest	Helpful in evaluating chest radiograph abnormalities
24-hour esophageal pH monitoring	May help link GERD and cough. Has a low specificity, so starting treatment for GERD may be preferable to testing as an initial decision
Barium esophagography	May reveal reflux in cases when refluxate from the stomach has a pH value similar to that of the normal esophagus, thus preventing its detection during esophageal pH monitoring.

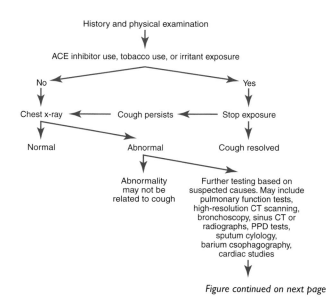

History and physical examination

ACE inhibitor use, tobacco use, or irritant exposure

No   Yes

Chest x-ray ← Cough persists ← Stop exposure

Normal   Abnormal   Cough resolved

Abnormality may not be related to cough

Further testing based on suspected causes. May include pulmonary function tests, high-resolution CT scanning, bronchoscopy, sinus CT or radiographs, PPD tests, sputum cylology, barium csophagography, cardiac studies

Figure continued on next page

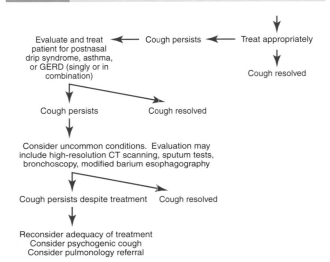

Figure 12-1. Evaluation of chronic cough in the immunocompetent host.

Further reading

Currie GP, Gray RD, McKay J. Chronic cough. British Medical Journal 2003;326: 261.

Holmes RL, Fadden CT. Evaluation of the patient with chronic cough. American Family Physician 2004;69: 2159–2166.

Irwin RS, Boulet IP, Cloutier MM, et al. Managing cough as a defense mechanism and as a symptom. A consensus panel report of the American College of Chest Physicians. Chest 1998;114(2 suppl managing): 166S.

Irwin RS, Madison JM. The diagnosis and treatment of cough. New England Journal of Medicine 2000;343: 1715–1721.

Irwin RS, Madison JM. The persistently troublesome cough. American Journal of Respiratory and Critical Care Medicine 2002;165: 1469–1474.

Lalloo UG, Barnes PJ, Chung KF. Pathophysiology and clinical presentations of cough. Journal of Allergy and Clinical Immunology 1996;98: 91S–96S.

Rosen MJ. Chronic cough due to tuberculosis and other infections: ACCP evidence-based clinical practice guidelines. Chest 2006;129: 197S–201S.

13 CHRONIC KIDNEY DISEASE

General Discussion

Chronic kidney disease (CKD) is defined by the presence of sustained abnormalities of renal function and results from different causes of renal injury. CKD can lead to progressive loss of renal function and may result in end-stage renal disease after a variable period of time following the initiating injury. The National Kidney Foundation has defined CKD as the presence of kidney damage for 3 or more months with or without decreased GFR. Kidney damage is manifested by pathologic abnormalities or markers of kidney damage, which include abnormalities in the composition of the blood or urine, such as proteinuria, abnormalities in the urine sediment, and abnormalities on imaging studies.

Among individuals with CKD, the stages are classified based on the level of kidney function.

- Stage 1   GFR ≥ 90
- Stage 2   GFR = 60–89
- Stage 3   GFR = 30–59
- Stage 4   GFR = 15–29
- Stage 5   GFR <15 or dialysis

Patients with CKD should be monitored for progression of renal failure. All individuals with GFR <60 for at least 3 months are classified as having CKD regardless of the presence or absence of kidney damage. When renal disease reaches this stage, the patient should be monitored more closely for control of hypertension, anemia, renal bone disease, and nutritional status.

Patients with CKD should be evaluated to determine the type of kidney disease, comorbid conditions, disease severity, complications, risk for loss of kidney function, and risk for development of cardiovascular disease.

Patients with CKD should be referred to a nephrologist for consultation and co-management if a clinical action plan cannot be prepared or the prescribed evaluation and recommended treatment cannot be carried out. In general, patients with GFR <30 mL/min/1.73 m^2 should be referred for nephrology consultation.

Risk Factors for Chronic Kidney Disease

Advancing age

Autoimmune diseases

Cardiovascular disease

Diabetes mellitus

Drug toxicity

Family history of kidney disease

Hyperlipidemia

Hypertension

Low birth weight

Low income/education

Lower urinary tract obstruction

Malignancy

Recovery from acute renal failure

Reduction in kidney mass

Smoking

Systemic infections

Urinary stones

Urinary tract infections

US ethnic minority status

- African-American
- Asian or Pacific Islander
- Hispanic
- Native American

Causes of Chronic Kidney Disease

Cystic diseases

- Polycystic kidney disease

Diabetic kidney disease

Glomerular diseases

- Autoimmune diseases
- Drugs
- Neoplasia
- Systemic infections

Transplant-related diseases

Tubulointerstitial diseases

- Drug toxicity
- Obstruction
- Stones
- Urinary tract infection

Vascular diseases

- Hypertension
- Large vessel disease
- Microangiopathy

Key Historical Features

✓ Symptoms during urination

✓ Recent infections

✓ Skin rash

✓ Arthritis

✓ Risk factors for HIV, hepatitis B, or hepatitis C

✓ Previous urologic evaluations

✓ Past medical history (hypertension, diabetes, heart failure, cirrhosis)

✓ Medications

✓ Family history of kidney diseases

Key Physical Findings

✓ Blood pressure

✓ Cardiovascular examination

✓ Skin examination for rash

✓ Joint examination for arthritis

Evaluation of Patients at Increased Risk of Chronic Kidney Disease

All patients:

Blood pressure measurement

Serum creatinine and estimate of GFR

Protein-to-creatinine ratio in a spot urine specimen

Examination of the urine sediment or dipstick for red blood cells and white blood cells

Evaluation of Patients with CKD

Serum creatinine and estimate of GFR

Protein-to-creatinine ratio in a spot urine specimen

Examination of the urine sediment or dipstick for red blood cells and white blood cells

Imaging of the kidneys, usually by ultrasound

Serum electrolytes

Clue	Potential Diagnosis
Review of Symptoms	
Symptoms during urination	Usually suggest disorders of the urinary tract such as infection, obstruction, or stones
Recent infections	May suggest post-infectious glomerulonephritis or HIV-associated nephropathy
Skin rash or arthritis	Suggests autoimmune disease, such as systemic lupus erythematosus or cryoglobulinemia
Risk factors for parenterally transmitted disease	May suggest HIV, hepatitis B or hepatitis C infection and associated kidney diseases
Chronic Diseases	
Heart failure, cirrhosis, or gastrointestinal fluid losses	Usually suggest reduced kidney perfusion ("pre-renal factors")
Diabetes*	As a cause of chronic kidney disease: diabetic kidney disease usually follows a typical clinical course after onset, first with microalbuminuria, followed by clinical proteinuria, hypertension, and declining GFR
Hypertension*	As a cause of chronic kidney disease: hypertensive nephrosclerosis is usually characterized by severely elevated blood pressure readings over a long period of time, with associated end-organ damage in addition to kidney disease. Recent worsening of hypertension, in association with findings of diffuse atherosclerosis, suggests large vessel disease due to atherosclerosis. Recent onset of severe hypertension in young women suggests large vessel disease due to fibromuscular dysplasia
Past Medical History	
Findings from past "routine" examinations	May reveal a history of hypertension or proteinuria during childhood, during pregnancy, or on examinations for school, military service, or insurance
Past urologic evaluations	Details may disclose radiologic abnormalities associated with kidney disease
Family History of Kidney Disease	
Every generation; equal susceptibility in males and females	Suggests an autosomal dominant disease, such as polycystic kidney disease
Every generation; predominant male susceptibility	Suggests a sex-linked recessive disease, such as Alport's syndrome
Less frequent than every generation	Suggests an autosomal recessive disease, such as medullary cystic kidney disease or autosomal recessive polycystic kidney disease

*Extremely common in elderly patients, and often nonspecific.

Table 13-1. Clues to the Diagnosis of Chronic Kidney Disease from the Patient's History

Disorder	Clinical clues	Urine sediment	Protein–creatinine ratio	Additional tests
Diabetes mellitus	Diabetes for >15 years, retinopathy	RBCs in <25% of affected patients	>30 to >3500 mg of protein per g of creatinine	Fasting blood sugar, A1C
Essential hypertension	Left ventricular hypertrophy, retinopathy	Benign	>30–3000 mg of protein per gram of creatinine	No additional tests
Glomerulonephritis	History and physical examination: infections; rash, arthritis; patient older than 40 years	Dysmorphic RBCs or RBC casts	>30 to >3500 mg of protein per g of creatinine	C3 and C4 for all patients Tests for infections: anti-ASO, ASK, HIV, HBsAg, HCV, RPR, blood cultures Tests if there is rash or arthritis: ANA, ANCA, cryoglobulin, anti-GBM Tests if patient is older than 40 years: SPEP, UPEP
Interstitial nephritis	Medications, fever, rash, eosinophilia	WBCs, WBC casts, eosinophils	30–3000 mg of protein per g of creatinine	ACE level; SS-A, SS-B
Low flow states	Volume depletion, hypotension, congestive heart failure, cirrhosis, atherosclerosis	Hyaline casts, eosinophils	<200 mg of protein per g of creatinine	FENa: <1% eosinophilia
Urinary tract obstruction	Urinary symptoms	Benign, or RBCs	None	KUB radiography, intravenous pyelography, spiral CT scanning, renal ultrasonography
Chronic urinary tract infection	Urinary symptoms	WBCs, RBCs	<2000 mg of protein per g of creatinine	Pelvic examination, urine culture, voiding cystourethrography, renal ultrasonography, CT scanning
Neoplasm, paraproteinemia	Patient older than 40 years, constitutional symptoms, anemia	RBCs, RBC casts, granular casts	False-negative result or >30 to >3500 mg of protein per g of creatinine	SPEP, UPEP, calcium level, ESR
Cystic kidney disease	Palpable kidneys with or without family history of cystic kidney disease, flank pain	RBCs	30–3000 mg of protein per g of creatinine	Renal ultrasonography or CT scanning if there is a complex kidney cyst or mass

Table 13-2. Diagnostic Evaluation in Chronic Kidney Disease

Continued

Disorder	Clinical clues	Urine sediment	Protein-creatinine ratio	Additional tests
Renovascular disease	Late-onset or refractory hypertension, sudden onset of hypertension in young woman, smoking history, abdominal bruit	Benign	<200 mg of protein per g of creatinine	Renal Doppler ultrasonography, radioisotope renal scanning, MRA, renal angiography
Vasculitis	Constitutional symptoms, peripheral neuropathy, rash, respiratory symptoms	RBCs; granular casts	>30 to >3500 mg of protein per g of creatinine	C3, C4, ANA, ANCA, HBsAg, HCV, cryoglobulins, ESR, RF, SS-A, SS-B, HIV

A1C = glycosylated hemoglobin; ACE = angiotensin-converting enzyme; ANA = antinuclear antibodies; ANCA = antineutrophil cytoplasmic antibody; anti-ASK = antistreptokinase; anti-GBM = anti-glomerular basement membrane antibody; ASO = streptolysin O latex antibody; C3 = complement 3; C4 = complement 4; CT = computed tomography; ESR = erythrocyte sedimentation rate; FENa = fractional excretion of sodium; HBsAg = hepatitis B surface antigen; HCV = hepatitis C virus; HIV = human immunodeficiency virus; KUB = kidney, ureters, and bladder; MRA = magnetic resonance angiography; RBC = red blood cell; RF = rheumatoid factor; RPR = rapid plasma reagin; SPEP = serum protein electrophoresis; SS-A = anti-Ro antibody; SS-B = anti-La antibody; UPEP = urine protein electrophoresis; WBC = white blood cell.

Adapted from Chronic kidney disease and pre-ESRD. Management in the primary care setting. Accessed February 24, 2005, at: http://www.oqp.med.va.gov/cpg/ESRD/ESRD_cpg/app/bot_app_1.htm.

Table 13-2. Diagnostic Evaluation in Chronic Kidney Disease

Additional Work-Up

The evaluation of the patient with CKD is guided by the symptoms, family history of kidney disease, medical history, physical exam findings, and findings from the urine sediment and protein-to-creatinine ratio.

Renal biopsy is indicated when the cause of CKD cannot be determined by the history and laboratory evaluation, or when the patient's signs and symptoms suggest renal parenchymal disease. Biopsy is more commonly required in patients with CKD that is not related to diabetes. Biopsy often is indicated in adult patients with nephrotic syndrome or suspected glomerulonephritis.

Further reading

Greenberg A, Cheung AK, National Kidney Foundation. Primer on kidney diseases, 3rd ed. San Diego: Academic Press; 2001.

Johnson CA, Levey AS, Coresh J, et al. Clinical practice guidelines for chronic kidney disease in adults: Part I: definition, disease stages, evaluation, treatment, and risk factors. American Family Physician 2004;70: 869–876.

Levin A, Stevens LA. Executing change in the management of chronic kidney disease: Perspectives on guidelines and practice. The Medical Clinics of North America 2005;89: 701–709.

McClellan WM. Epidemiology and risk factors for chronic kidney disease. The Medical Clinics of North America 2005;89: 419–445.

National Kidney Foundation. K/DOQI clinical practice guidelines for chronic kidney disease: evaluation, classification, and stratification. Online. Available: http://www.kidney.org/professionals/kdoqi/guidelines_ckd/toc.htm 16 May 2006.

Snyder S, Pendergraph B. Detection and evaluation of chronic kidney disease. American Family Physician 2005;72: 1723–1732.

14 CHRONIC MENINGITIS

General Discussion

Meningitis can be divided based on time course, associated CSF profile, and underlying cause. Chronic meningitis is arbitrarily defined as meningitis that persists for 4 or more weeks. It is important to document that patients are not in a slow recovery phase as this distinguishes them from resolving acute meningitis cases.

Chronic meningitis is uncommon and accounts for less than 10% of all meningitis cases. It has the widest spectrum of causes and occurs in both immunocompetent and immunocompromised individuals. Chronic meningitis may be caused by many different pathogens as well as by noninfectious causes. The major infectious causes are tuberculous meningitis and cryptococcal meningitis. The major noninfectious causes are neoplastic disease, neurosarcoidosis, and vasculitis.

The CSF examination is helpful in differentiating the patient with chronic meningitis from the patient with acute meningitis, encephalitis, or recurrent meningitis. A mildly decreased glucose in the setting of mononuclear pleocytosis should raise the possibility of chronic meningitis.

Causes of Chronic Meningitis

Bacterial

- Mycobacterial (*M. tuberculosis*, *M. avium*)
- Spirochetal (*Borrelia burgdorferi*, *Leptospira interrogans*, *Treponema pallidum*)
- *Agents causing sinus tracts (Actinomycetes, Arachnia, Nocardia)*
- *Brucella*
- *Tropheryma whippelii*
- *L. monocytogenes*
- *N. meningitides*
- *Francisella tularensis*

Fungal

- *Cryptococcus neoformans*
- *Coccidioides immitis*
- *Histoplasma capsulatum*
- *Candida* sp.
- Other mycoses (*Aspergillus*, *Blastomyces*, *Dematiaceous* sp, *Paracoccidioides*, *Pseudallescheria*, *Sporothrix*, *Trichosporon beigelii*, *Zygomycetes*)

Parasitic

- *Taenia solium* (cysticercosis)
- *Acanthamoeba*
- *Angiostrongylus*
- *Toxoplasma gondii*
- *Coenurus cerebralis*
- *Schistosoma* sp.

Viral

- Retroviruses (HIV-1, HTLV-1)
- Enteroviruses
- Herpesvirus

Noninfectious

- Neoplastic
- Neurosarcoidosis
- Vasculitis
- Behçet's disease
- Chemical meningitis
- Fabry's disease
- Hypertrophic pachymeningitis
- Systemic lupus erythematosus
- Uveomeningoencephalitides

Idiopathic

- Chronic benign lymphocytic meningitis

Key Historical Features

✓ Fever

✓ Headache

✓ Stiff neck

✓ Nausea and vomiting

✓ Photophobia

✓ Drowsiness

✓ Malaise

✓ Chronicity of symptoms

✓ Previous systemic infections (tuberculosis, fungal infection, syphilis)

✓ Past medical history, especially malignancy, autoimmune disease, systemic vasculitis, or immunocompromised status

✓ Travel history

✓ Geographic risk factors

✓ Animal exposures

✓ Work exposures

Key Physical Findings

✓ Vital signs

✓ Funduscopic examination for papilledema

✓ Ophthalmologic examination for eye lesions

✓ Neck examination for meningismus

✓ Lymph node examination for lymphadenopathy

✓ Dermatologic examination for skin lesions

✓ General examination for evidence of infection or systemic disease

✓ Neurologic examination

Suggested Work-Up for Chronic Meningitis (not all are necessary in all cases)

Blood tests

- Complete blood count with differential
- Serum chemistries
- Erythrocyte sedimentation rate
- Antinuclear antibodies
- HIV serology
- Rapid plasma reagin (RPR)
- Consider angiotensin-converting enzyme (ACE), antineutrophilic cytoplasmic antibodies, specific serologies, blood smears

CSF

- Cell count with differential, protein, glucose
- Cytology
- Venereal Disease Research Laboratory (VDRL)
- Cultures (TB, fungal, bacterial, viral)
- Stain (Gram, acid fast, India ink)
- Cryptococcal antigen
- Oligoclonal bands, IgG index
- Consider ACE; PCR (viruses, mycobacteria, *T. whippelii*); histoplasma antigen, immunocytochemistry (*T. whippelii* and other selected agents); paired antibodies for *B. burgdorferi*, *Brucella*, histoplasma, *Coccidioides*, other fungal agents; neoplastic markers

Neuroimaging

- Brain MR imaging with contrast
- Consider CT, spinal MR imaging, angiography

Cultures

- Blood (parasites, fungi, viruses, rare bacteria)
- Urine (mycobacteria, viruses, fungi)
- Sputum (mycobacteria, fungi)
- Consider gastric washings, stool, bone marrow, liver (mycobacteria, fungi)

Ancillary

- Chest radiograph
- Electrocardiogram
- Selected testing (mammogram, CT chest/abdomen)

Biopsy

- Extraneural sites (bone marrow, lymph node, peripheral nerve, liver, lung, skin, small bowel)

Useful Serologic Tests in the Chronic Meningitis Syndrome

Bacteria

- *B. burgdorferi*
- *Brucella*
- *Leptospira*
- *Treponema pallidum* (RPR, VDRL)

Fungi

- *Aspergillus* sp.
- *Coccidioides immitis*
- *Histoplasma capsulatum*
- *Sporothrix schenckii*
- *Zygomycetes*

Parasites

- *Taenia solium*
- *Toxoplasma gondii*

Viruses

- HIV-1
- HTLV-1

Further reading

Coyle PK. Overview of acute and chronic meningitis. Neurologic Clinics 1999;17: 691–710.
Goetz C. Textbook of clinical neurology, 2nd ed. Philadelphia: Saunders; 2003:511–524.

General Discussion

A complaint of constipation may mean very different things to different patients. A complaint of constipation may mean infrequent bowel movements, straining while stooling, incomplete evacuation, abdominal pain, abdominal bloating, hard stools, small stools, or a need for digital manipulation to enable defecation. An international committee has recommended definitions of chronic functional constipation.

The Rome II criteria for functional constipation are two or more of the following symptoms for at least 12 weeks in the past 12 months:

- Straining in more than 1 out of 4 defecations
- Lumpy or hard stool in more than 1 out of 4 defecations
- Sensation of incomplete evacuation in more than 1 out of 4 defecations
- Sensation of anorectal obstruction or blockage in more than 1 out of 4 defecations
- Manual maneuvers to facilitate more than 1 out of 4 defecations
- Fewer than three bowel movements per week
- Loose stools are not present and there is insufficient criteria for irritable bowel syndrome

There are a wide variety of potential causes of constipation, and the majority of individuals with constipation do not have an identifiable cause to explain their symptoms. Constipation may occur due to an alteration in stool consistency, stool caliber, or colonic motility. Constipation also may result from a change in the process of rectal evacuation, usually due to an obstruction of the movement of luminal contents or poor colonic propulsive activity. It is important to distinguish functional constipation from other disorders that may be associated with altered bowel habits. The evaluation of constipation aims to exclude systemic disease or a structural disorder of the intestines.

Medications Associated with Constipation

Adrenergic agents

Aluminum antacids

Anticholinergics

Anticonvulsants

Antihistamines

Antiparkinson drugs

Antipsychotics

Antispasmodics

Barium sulfate

Beta blockers

Calcium

Calcium channel blockers

Diuretics

Iron supplements

NSAIDs

Opioids

Sucralfate

Tricyclic antidepressants

Causes of Constipation

Adhesions

Amyloidosis

Anorexia nervosa

Autonomic neuropathy

Bulimia nervosa

Cerebrovascular disease

Colorectal cancer

Congenital megacolon (Hirschsprung's disease)

Depression

Dermatomyositis

Diabetes mellitus

External compression

Heavy metal poisoning

Hirschsprung's disease

Hypercalcemia

Hypokalemia

Hypomagnesemia

Hypopituitarism

Hypothyroidism

Inflammatory stricture

- • Diverticulitis
- • Inflammatory bowel disease
- • Postischemic injury

Irritable bowel syndrome (constipation-predominant type)

Leiomyoma

Lipoma

Medications

Multiple sclerosis

Muscular dystrophies

Myopathy

Myotonic dystrophy

Neurofibromatosis

Neuropathy

- Aganglionosis
- Hyperganglionosis
- Chagas disease
- Idiopathic
- Paraneoplastic

Parkinson's disease

Pelvic floor weakness

Pelvic outlet obstruction

Pheochromocytoma

Porphyria

Pregnancy

Primary functional constipation

- Slow-transit constipation
- Pelvic floor dysfunction

Rectocele

Shy Drager syndrome

Spinal cord injury

Systemic sclerosis

Uremia

Key Historical Features

✓ Size, consistency, and frequency of the bowel movements

✓ Onset and duration of the symptoms

✓ Red flag symptoms

- Weight loss
- Melena
- Rectal bleeding
- Changes in bowel habits or stool caliber
- Fever

- • Abdominal pain or cramping
- • Nausea or vomiting
- • Rectal pain
✓ Dietary habits and fluid intake
✓ Bowel habits
✓ History of fecal incontinence
✓ Work habits
✓ Level of physical activity
✓ Medical history
✓ Surgical and obstetrical history
✓ Medications
✓ Laxative and vitamin use

Key Physical Findings

✓ Vital signs
✓ Abdominal examination for bowel sounds, masses, distention, tenderness, organomegaly, and surgical scars
✓ Anorectal examination and anocutaneous reflex
✓ Color and consistency of the stool
✓ Detailed neurologic examination
✓ Body hair and skin examination for signs of hypothyroidism
✓ Signs of depression or anxiety

Suggested Work-Up

CBC	To evaluate for malignancy or infection
TSH	To evaluate for hypothyroidism
Calcium	To evaluate for hypercalcemia
Glucose	To evaluate for diabetes mellitus
Electrolytes	To evaluate for hypokalemia
Magnesium	To evaluate for hypomagnesemia
BUN and creatinine	To evaluate for renal disease

Stool for occult blood	To help evaluate for gastrointestinal malignancy
Colonoscopy or barium enema and flexible sigmoidoscopy	To rule out lesions that narrow the bowel in adults with constipation and iron-deficiency anemia, a positive stool guaiac test, or a first-degree relative with colon cancer

Additional Work-Up

Abdominal radiographs	Can detect retained stool and suggest evidence of impaction or volvulus
Serum protein electrophoresis and urine protein electrophoresis	If multiple myeloma is suspected
Anorectal manometry	To assess the anal sphincter, pelvic floor, and associated nerves. Helps to exclude Hirschsprung's disease
Balloon insertion	To help rule out pelvic floor dysfunction
Defecography	For patients with intractable constipation or pelvic floor disorders to evaluate evacuatory disorders such as rectal prolapse and rectocele
Colonic transit studies	To evaluate the rate of colonic transit and to rule out pelvic outlet obstruction

Further reading

Arce DA, Ermocilla CA, Costa H. Evaluation of constipation. American Family Physician 2002;65: 2283–2290.

Borum ML. Constipation: evaluation and management. Primary Care Clinics in Office Practice 2001;28: 577–590.

Faigel DO. A clinical approach to constipation. Clinical Cornerstone 2002;4: 11–21.

Rao SSC. Constipation: evaluation and treatment. Gastroenterology Clinics of North America 2003;32: 659–683.

Thompson WG, Longstreth GF, Drossman DA, et al. Functional bowel disorders and functional abdominal pain. Gut 1999;45(Suppl II): 43–47.

16 DELIRIUM

General Discussion

Delirium is an acute disturbance in mental status characterized by fluctuating levels of consciousness and an impairment of attention. Fluctuations in cognitive skills such as memory, language, and organization are common. In general, any patient with acute onset of confusion or mental deterioration should be considered to be delirious until another diagnosis is found. The following is a list of the DSM-IV criteria for delirium:

- Disturbance of consciousness (e.g., reduced clarity of awareness about the environment) with reduced ability to focus, sustain, or shift attention.

- A change in cognition (e.g., memory deficit, disorientation, language disturbance) or development of a perceptual disturbance that is not better accounted for by a preexisting, established, or evolving dementia.

- The disturbance develops over a short period of time (usually hours to days) and tends to fluctuate during the course of a day.

- Evidence from the history, physical examination, or laboratory findings indicates that the disturbance is caused by direct physiologic consequences of a general medical condition.

The three subtypes of delirium are hyperactive, hypoactive, and mixed. Patients with the hyperactive subtype may demonstrate restlessness, anxiety, sleep disturbances, irritability, increased psychomotor activity, emotional lability, anger, and euphoria. The presentation of the hyperactive subtype may mimic schizophrenia, psychotic disorder, or agitated dementia.

Patients with the hypoactive subtype may demonstrate reduced attention, altered arousal, decreased psychomotor activity, sadness, and disorientation. The mixed subtype is characterized by fluctuations between the hyperactive and hypoactive subtypes.

Other clinical features of delirium include delusions, hallucinations, disorganized thinking, incoherent speech, memory impairment, and disorientation to time, place, or person. Neurologic abnormalities may be present, including dysgraphia, tremor, myoclonus, reflex changes, and tone changes.

Delirium is often initially misdiagnosed as depression or dementia. In distinguishing delirium from depression, an evaluation of the onset and timeline of depressive and cognitive symptoms is important. The degree of cognitive impairment in delirium is much more severe and pervasive than in depression, with a more abrupt temporal onset. In addition, delirium manifests a disturbance in arousal or consciousness, while it is usually not a feature of depression. When considering dementia, it is important to remember that the patient with dementia is alert and does not have the disturbance of consciousness or arousal that is characteristic of delirium. Dementia is characterized by a more gradual onset of symptoms and is chronically progressive, with less impairment of the sleep–wake cycle.

Despite advances in medical technology, the cornerstone in the evaluation of delirium remains the history and physical examination. After a thorough evaluation, laboratory testing and diagnostic imaging may be warranted but should be individualized on a case-by-case basis. It may be helpful to keep in mind the five leading causes of delirium: (1) fluid/ electrolyte disturbances, (2) infection, (3) medication toxicity, (4) metabolic derangement, and (5) sensory and environmental disturbance.

Medications Associated with Delirium

Antiarrhythmics
- Amiodarone
- Disopyramide
- Quinidine

Anticholinergic agents

Antiemetics

Anticonvulsant agents
- Carbamazepine
- Phenytoid

Antihistamines

Antihypertensives
- Methyldopa
- Propranolol
- Reserpine

Antiparkinson drugs
- Amantadine
- Bromocriptine
- Levodopa/carbidopa
- Pergolide

Antipsychotic agents

Aspirin

Benzodiazepines
- Diazepam
- Lorazepam
- Temazepam

Benztropine

Beta blockers

Calcium channel blockers

Chemotherapeutic agents

- Asparaginase
- Bleomycin
- Carmustine
- Cisplatin
- Fluorouracil
- Procarbazine
- Methotrexate
- Vinblastine
- Vincristine

Cold remedies

Corticosteroids

Cyclosporine

Diphenhydramine

Digoxin

Diuretics

Gastrointestinal antispasmodics

Histamine$_2$-receptor blockers

- Cimetidine
- Famotidine
- Nizatidine
- Ranitidine

Hypoglycemic agents

- Glimepiride
- Glipizide
- Glyburide

Ipratropium (inhaled)

Lithium

Metoclopramide

Narcotics

- Hydromorphone
- Levorphanol
- Meperidine
- Morphine sulfate

NSAIDs

Oxybutynin

Sleep aids

Tricyclic antidepressants

Causes of Delirium

Anemia

Cardiovascular disease

- Acute myocardial infarction
- Arrhythmia
- Congestive heart failure
- Hypertensive encephalopathy
- Hypotension

Fluid and electrolyte disturbances

- Dehydration
- Hypercalcemia
- Hyperkalemia
- Hypernatremia
- Hypocalcemia
- Hypokalemia
- Hypomagnesemia
- Hyponatremia
- Hypotension

Hepatic disease

- Hepatic insufficiency

Infection

- Bacteremia
- Cholecystitis
- Diverticulitis
- Encephalitis
- Herpes zoster
- HIV infection
- Meningitis
- Pneumonia
- Sepsis
- Tetanus
- Tuberculosis
- Urinary tract infection

Malignancy and paraneoplastic syndromes

Medications

Metabolic abnormalities

- Hypoglycemia
- Hypoxia
- Parathyroid dysfunction
- Renal insufficiency
- Thyroid dysfunction
- Vitamin deficiencies

Neurologic disease

- Cerebral vasculitis
- Cerebrovascular accident
- Seizure
- Subdural hematoma (acute and chronic)
- Temporal arteritis

Pulmonary disease

- Pulmonary embolism

Toxins

- Alcohol
- Drugs

Withdrawal syndromes

- Alcohol
- Benzodiazepines
- Other sedatives

Key Historical Features

✓ Patient age

✓ Premorbid condition and functional level

- Occupation
- Level of alertness
- Ability for self-care
- Intellectual activity

✓ History of present illness

- Onset
- Rate of symptom development
- Course over the last 24 hours
- Patient's physical complaints
- Recent falls or head trauma

✓ Past medical history

✓ Past surgical history, especially recent surgery

✓ Medications

✓ Over-the-counter medications, herbal remedies, and supplements

✓ Substance use (alcohol, tobacco, recreational drugs)

Key Physical Findings

✓ Vital signs

✓ Pulse oximetry

✓ Funduscopic exam

✓ Head, eyes, ears, nose, throat (HEENT) exam for dilated pupils or flushing

✓ Cardiovascular exam

✓ Pulmonary exam

✓ Abdominal exam for evidence of gastrointestinal pathology

✓ Evidence of trauma, metabolic disturbance, dehydration, or sepsis

✓ Neurologic exam for focal deficits, asterixis, tremor, myoclonus, or evidence of CNS infection

✓ Mini-mental status exam

Suggested Work-Up

Mini mental status exam	To assess cognitive status
Complete blood count (CBC)	To assess for infection or anemia
Electrolytes	To evaluate for sodium or potassium disturbances
BUN and creatinine	To assess renal function
Blood glucose	To evaluate for hypo- or hyperglycemia
Calcium	To evaluate for calcium disturbances
AST, ALT, and albumin	To evaluate for hepatic abnormalities
Urinalysis	To evaluate for urinary tract infection

Chest X-ray	To evaluate for pulmonary infection or cardiopulmonary disease
EKG	For elderly patients or patients with a cardiac history or cardiac risk factors
Head CT or MRI	For patients with a history of falls, suspected trauma, or focal neurologic findings

Additional Work-Up

EEG	May be used to differentiate delirium from other conditions and to rule out ictal and postictal seizure activity (delirium demonstrates a diffuse slowing of the background rhythm)
Creatine phosphokinase	If acute myocardial infarction is suspected
Erythrocyte sedimentation rate	If vasculitis, inflammatory, or rheumatologic condition is suspected
Lumbar puncture/CSF fluid examination	For febrile patients when meningitis or encephalitis is suspected
Toxicology screening	When toxin exposure is suspected
Levels of prescribed drugs	For appropriate drugs in which elevated levels may cause delirium
Arterial blood gas	To further evaluate hypoxia or acid/base disturbances

Further reading

Breitbart W, Strout D. Delirium in the terminally ill. Clinics in Geriatric Medicine 2000; 16: 357–372.

Diagnostic and statistical manual of mental disorders: DSM-IV-TR. Washington, D.C.: American Psychiatric Association; 2000.

Gleason OC. Delirium. American Family Physician 2003;67: 1027–1034.

Jacobson SA. Delirium in the elderly. Psychiatric Clinics of North America 1997;20: 91–110.

Marsh CM. Psychiatric presentations of medical illness. Psychiatric Clinics of North America 1997;20: 181–204.

Murphy BA. Delirium. Emergency Medicine Clinics of North America 2000;18: 243–252.

Winawer N. Postoperative delirium. Medical Clinics of North America 2001;85: 1229–1239.

17 DEMENTIA AND MEMORY LOSS

General Discussion

Dementia is a common syndrome among older persons and is characterized by the gradual onset and continuing decline of higher cognitive functioning. Dementia becomes more prevalent in each decade of life, affecting approximately 1% to 10% of adults 65 years old and 50% of those older than 90 years of age.

Dementia should be suspected when there is an impairment in memory and an impairment of at least one other domain of higher cognitive functioning that interferes with normal social and executive functioning in an otherwise alert person. These domains include judgment, abstract thinking, complex task performance, apraxia, agnosia, visuospatial awareness, and personality change. These changes are present without other significant neurologic signs or symptoms (parkinsonism or focal neurologic signs), psychiatric disease, or systemic illnesses (such as thyroid deficiency, vitamin deficiencies, or chronic infections).

Early symptoms may be present that can suggest the presence of a dementing illness. These symptoms include difficulty in learning and retaining new information, difficulty performing complex tasks, altered reasoning, problems with spatial awareness (getting lost in familiar places), difficulties with language (difficulty expressing oneself or difficulty following conversations), and behavioral changes (such as becoming more irritable, suspicious, or aggressive than usual).

Depression is common in the elderly and should be considered in any patient being evaluated for dementia. Patients with neurologic disorders that cause dementia, such as stroke and Alzheimer's dementia, may be more prone to associated depression.

Common Causes of Dementia

Alzheimer's dementia

Vascular dementia

Mixed dementia

Other

- Depression
- Frontotemporal dementia
- Parkinson's disease
- Alcohol-related dementia
- Huntington's disease
- Prion disease
- Trauma

- Chronic infections (neurosyphilis, AIDS)
- Encephalitis
- Hypothyroidism
- Vitamin B_{12} deficiency

Suggested Work-Up

TSH	To evaluate for hypothyroidism
Vitamin B_{12}	To evaluate for vitamin B_{12} deficiency
CBC	To evaluate for chronic infection
Electrolytes	To evaluate for metabolic derangement
Calcium	To evaluate for hypercalcemia
Glucose	To evaluate for hypoglycemia and diabetes
MRI or noncontrast CT of the brain	Recommended by the American Academy of Neurology for all patients as part of the initial evaluation of dementia

Additional Work-Up

The following tests should be performed when clinical suspicion warrants them.

RPR	To evaluate for syphilis
Lyme disease titer	To evaluate for Lyme disease
HIV	To evaluate for HIV/AIDS and possible opportunistic infections
Urinalysis, urine culture and sensitivity	To evaluate for urinary tract infection
Erythrocyte sedimentation rate	To evaluate for inflammatory diseases
AST, ALT, bilirubin	To evaluate for liver disease
Folic acid	To evaluate for folic acid deficiency

Heavy metal assays	To evaluate for exposure to heavy metals
Lumbar puncture	Should be considered for patients with suspected cerebral vasculitis, HIV infection, neurosyphilis, prion disease, or cerebral Lyme disease
Neuropsychologic testing	Can comprehensively assess multiple domains of higher cognitive functioning including intelligence and behavioral functioning and can be used to identify cognitive impairment in patients with higher baseline cognitive abilities. It may also reveal subtle cognitive impairment in persons with suspected cognitive impairment or dementia. Neuropsychologic testing is not recommended routinely for all patients with suspected dementia
Electroencephalography	Indicated only if prion disease is suspected

Further reading

Adelman AM, Daly MP. Initial evaluation of the patient with suspect dementia. American Family Physician 2005; 71: 1745–1750.

Diagnostic and statistical manual of mental disorders, 4th ed. Washington D.C.: American Psychiatric Association; 2000.

Friedland RP, Wilcock GK. Dementia. In: Evans JG, Williams TF, Beattie BL, Michel JP, Wilcock GK, eds. Oxford textbook of geriatric medicine, 2nd ed. Oxford: Oxford University Press; 2000:922–932.

Kaye JA. Diagnostic challenges in dementia. Neurology 1998;51: S45–S52.

Knopman DS, DeKosky ST, Cummings JL, et al. Practice parameter: diagnosis of dementia (an evidence-based review). Neurology 2001;56: 1143–1153.

Leifer BP. Early diagnosis of Alzheimer's disease; clinical and economic benefits. Journal of the American Geriatrics Society 2003;51:(5 suppl Dementia): S281–S288.

18 DIARRHEA

General Discussion

Diarrhea is a change in stools, usually defined clinically as the passage of 3 or more loose or watery stools or 1 or more bloody stool in 24 hours. Acute diarrhea lasts less than 14 days, persistent diarrhea lasts more than 14 days, and chronic diarrhea lasts more than 1 month.

Patients who present with acute diarrhea are more likely to have an infectious cause. Patients with chronic diarrhea have a much broader group of diagnoses to consider. The list below provides an outline of most causes for diarrhea. Most cases of acute diarrhea are self-limited and do not require further evaluation. Indications for stool studies in acute diarrhea include fever, bloody diarrhea, history of travel to an endemic area, recent antibiotic use, a history of inflammatory bowel disease, exposure to infants in day care centers, and a history of anal intercourse. If the patient does not meet these criteria but the diarrhea persists for more than a few days, a more detailed evaluation is warranted.

The medical history is the key to the evaluation of most patients presenting with diarrhea and can help guide the diagnostic work-up. Important historical features are outlined below.

Medications That May Cause Diarrhea

Antacids containing calcium or magnesium

Antibiotics

Colchicine

Enteral tube feeds

Laxatives

Sorbitol gums (acarbose)

Causes of Diarrhea

Bacteria

- Aeromonas
- Campylobacter
- *Clostridium difficile*
- Enterotoxigenic *E. coli*
- Other *E. coli*
- Salmonella (non-typhoid)
- Shigella
- Tuberculosis
- Vibrio (non-cholera)

Congenital syndromes

Diabetic autonomic neuropathy

Diverticulitis

Endocrine causes

- Addison's disease
- Carcinoid syndrome
- Gastrinoma
- Hyperthyroidism
- Mastocytosis
- Medullary carcinoma of the thyroid
- Somatostatinoma
- VIPoma

Ileal bile acid malabsorption

Inflammatory bowel disease

Intestinal ischemia

Irritable bowel syndrome

Malabsorption syndromes

- Carbohydrate malabsorption
- Celiac disease
- Short bowel syndrome

Malignancy

- Colon cancer
- Lymphoma

Medications

Other

- Mixed infection

Pancreatic exocrine insufficiency

Parasites

- Cryptosporidium
- Cyclospora
- Entamoeba histolytica
- Giardia
- Isospora belli
- Schistosoma
- Strongyloides
- Trichuris

Postsympathectomy diarrhea

Postvagotomy diarrhea

Radiation

Vasculitis

Viruses

- Cytomegalovirus
- Herpes simplex
- Toroviruses
- Rotavirus

Key Historical Features

✓ Onset of illness

✓ Duration of symptoms

✓ Quantification of diarrhea

✓ Characterization of the stools

✓ Presence of blood in the stools

✓ Weight loss

✓ Presence of nocturnal diarrhea

✓ Presence of other gastrointestinal symptoms

- Nausea and vomiting
- Abdominal pain
- Fever
- Fecal urgency

✓ Volume status

- Thirst
- Dizziness
- Urination
- Syncope

✓ Travel to endemic areas

✓ Exposure to untreated water

✓ Medication use (especially antibiotics or laxatives)

✓ Medical history, including history of radiation

✓ Surgical history

✓ Occupational exposures

✓ Immune status

✓ Sexual preference

✓ Dietary history

Key Physical Findings

✓ Vital signs
- Fever
- Tachycardia
- Postural hypotension

✓ Findings of dehydration
- Mucous membranes
- Capillary refill
- Skin turgor

✓ Abdominal examination (rule out peritoneal signs)

✓ Rectal examination
- Stool character
- Presence of blood

Suggested Work-Up for Acute or Persistent Diarrhea

CBC	To evaluate for an elevated white blood cell count, anemia, or hemoconcentration
Serum electrolytes	To evaluate for electrolyte disturbance
BUN and creatinine	To evaluate for volume depletion or acute renal failure
Stool evaluation for white blood cells	To evaluate for infection
Abdominal radiographs	In toxic patients to help confirm the diagnosis of colitis and to look for evidence of ileus or megacolon

Additional Work-Up for Acute or Persistent Diarrhea

Stool evaluation for ova and parasites	If a parasitic infection is suspected
Stool culture	If fecal white blood cells are positive
Ameba serology	If amebiasis is suspected
Giardia antigen	If Giardia infection is suspected

Clostridium difficile toxin assay in stool specimen	If the patient has been on antibiotics in the preceding 3 months or if a patient develops diarrhea in an institutional setting
Sigmoidoscopy	May be considered in toxic patients, patients with blood in the stool, or patients with persistent diarrhea
Colonoscopy	In AIDS patients with diarrhea to rule out infection or lymphoma in the ascending colon

Suggested Work-Up for Chronic Diarrhea

The work-up for acute or persistent diarrhea should be considered in addition to the work-up outlined below.

Stool sodium and potassium concentrations	To calculate an osmotic gap in stool water
Stool pH	To help detect carbohydrate malabsorption
Fecal occult blood testing	To help detect colitis or malignancy
Assessment for stool white blood cells	To evaluate for infection
Fecal fat concentration	To help detect pancreatic exocrine insufficiency. Steatorrhea suggests dysfunction of absorption by the small intestine
Laxative screen	To detect laxative ingestion

Additional Work-Up for Chronic Diarrhea

TSH	To evaluate for thyroid disease if it is suspected clinically
Blood glucose	To evaluate for diabetes mellitus if it is suspected

CT scan of the abdomen	To help detect small bowel disease, colonic disease, and pancreatic tumors
Sigmoidoscopy or colonoscopy	To evaluate for inflammatory bowel disease and tumors. Also allows biopsy to be performed.
Stool magnesium level	If magnesium ingestion is suspected

Further reading

Gore JI, Surawicz C. Severe acute diarrhea. Gastroenterology Clinics of North America 2003;32: 1249–1267.

Lee SD, Surawicz CM. Infectious causes of chronic diarrhea. Gastroenterology Clinics 2001;30:679–692.

Schiller LR. Diarrhea. Advances in Gastroenterology 2000;84: 1259–1274.

Schiller L, Sellin J. Diarrhea. In: Feldman LF, Sleisenger M, eds. Gastrointestinal and liver disease, vol. 1, 7th ed. Philadelphia: WB Saunders; 2002.

Yates J. Traveler's diarrhea. American Family Physician 2005;71: 2095–2100.

General Discussion

In its consensus statement, the American Thoracic Society has defined dyspnea as "a subjective experience of breathing discomfort that consists of qualitatively distinct sensations that vary in intensity." The experience of dyspnea derives from interactions among multiple physiological, psychological, social, and environmental factors. One of the more popular theories of dyspnea states that dyspnea results from a disassociation or a mismatch between central respiratory motor activity and incoming afferent information from receptors in the airways, lungs, and chest wall structures. The development of shortness of breath is an expected outcome of overexertion, such as occurs after running or heavy lifting. However, when dyspnea occurs at rest or during exertion that is less than expected, it is considered pathologic and a symptom of a disease state.

Many patients have a likely cause of dyspnea, such as exacerbation of known congestive heart failure, chronic obstructive pulmonary disease (COPD), or asthma. However, in others the diagnosis may not be readily apparent even after a thorough history and physical examination. The first step in the evaluation of the patient with dyspnea is to determine the status of the patient: (1) distress with unstable vital signs; (2) distress with stable vital signs; or (3) no distress and stable vital signs. The next step in the evaluation of patients with dyspnea is to establish the primary organ system involved: pulmonary, cardiac, both, or neither.

In the elderly patient, dyspnea is generally due to one of five major etiologies: (1) cardiac disease, (2) respiratory disease, (3) deconditioning/obesity, (4) respiratory muscle dysfunction, or (5) psychological disorders. The patient's age, comparison with peers, daily or usual activities, overall fitness level, and any other medical problems must be considered.

In most patients, the cause or causes of dyspnea can be determined by using the history and physical examination to identify common etiologies, particularly cardiac and pulmonary causes. In some cases, specific diagnostic testing or consultation may be required to establish or confirm the diagnosis.

Medications Associated with Dyspnea

Amiodarone (pneumonitis)

Aspirin overdose

Beta blockers (may aggravate obstructive airway disease)

Nitrofurantoin (pneumonitis)

Causes of Dyspnea

Cardiac causes

- Arrhythmia
- Asymmetric septal hypertrophy
- Congestive heart failure
- Coronary artery disease
- Myocardial infarction
- Pericardial disease
- Valvular disease

Metabolic and endocrine causes

- Carbon monoxide poisoning
- Metabolic acidosis
- Salicylate poisoning
- Thyroid disease
- Uremia

Medications

Neuromuscular causes

- Amyotrophic lateral sclerosis
- Guillain–Barré syndrome
- Myasthenia gravis

Psychogenic causes

- Anxiety
- Depression
- Hyperventilation
- Panic attacks
- Post-traumatic stress disorder
- Secondary gain/malingering
- Somatization disorder

Pulmonary causes

- Asbestosis
- Aspiration (may be due to gastroesophageal reflux disease)
- Asthma
- Berylliosis
- Bronchiectasis
- COPD
- Coal workers' lung
- Hypersensitivity pneumonitis
- Malignancy (primary or metastatic)
- Pleural effusion

- Pleural thickening
- Pneumoconiosis
- Pneumonia
- Pneumothorax
- Pulmonary edema
- Pulmonary embolism
- Pulmonary hypertension
- Restrictive lung disease
- Silicosis

Upper airway obstruction

- Croup
- Epiglottitis
- Foreign body aspiration
- Laryngeal disease
- Tracheal stenosis
- Vocal cord paralysis

Other causes

- Abdominal mass
- Anemia
- Aspirin overdose
- Chest wall deformities
- Deconditioning
- Food allergy
- Liver cirrhosis
- Obesity
- Opportunistic infection in an immunosuppressed patient
- Pain
- Thoracic burn with eschar formation
- Trauma

Key Historical Features

✓ Onset

✓ Duration

✓ Frequency

✓ Descriptive qualities

✓ Intensity

- ✓ Triggers
- ✓ Relieving factors
- ✓ Occurrence at rest or with exertion
- ✓ Orthopnea
- ✓ Paroxysmal nocturnal dyspnea
- ✓ Wheezing
- ✓ Edema
- ✓ Presence of cough or sputum production
- ✓ Fever
- ✓ Chest pain, radiation of pain, nausea, or diaphoresis
- ✓ Leg swelling, redness, warmth, or pain
- ✓ Sore throat
- ✓ Indigestion
- ✓ Dysphagia
- ✓ Hemoptysis
- ✓ Anxiety symptoms
- ✓ History of trauma
- ✓ History of scuba diving
- ✓ Past medical history, especially heart disease
- ✓ Past surgical history, especially recent surgery
- ✓ Medications
- ✓ Family history
- ✓ Smoking history and exposure to secondhand smoke
- ✓ Occupational exposures to asbestos, dust, or volatile chemicals

Key Physical Findings

- ✓ Vital signs
- ✓ Body weight to compare with previous values
- ✓ General appearance, mental status, ability to speak
- ✓ Observation of breathing pattern and use of accessory muscles
- ✓ Neck examination for distended neck veins, thyroid enlargement, tracheal position, and stridor

✓ Chest examination for dullness to percussion, subcutaneous emphysema, or kyphoscoliosis

✓ Cardiac examination for heart rate, murmurs, or extra heart sounds

✓ Pulmonary examination for breath sounds, wheezing, or rales

✓ Abdominal examination for hepatomegaly, masses, ascites, or hepatojugular reflux

✓ Extremity examination for edema or evidence of deep venous thrombosis. Digit examination for cyanosis or clubbing

Suggested Work-Up

Pulse oximetry	To determine oxygenation level. Useful to measure at rest and after exercise
Chest radiograph	To evaluate for conditions such as congestive heart failure, pulmonary edema, pneumonia, pneumothorax, or COPD
Electrocardiogram	To evaluate for ischemia, arrhythmia, or left ventricular hypertrophy
Spirometry	To distinguish obstructive lung disorders from restrictive lung disorders
CBC	To evaluate for anemia, infection, or erythrocytosis
Electrolytes, BUN, creatinine, magnesium, and calcium	To evaluate for acid–base disturbances, intravascular volume disturbances, electrolyte abnormalities, or uremia

Additional Work-Up

Echocardiogram	To evaluate for heart failure, ventricular hypertrophy, valvular dysfunction, or elevated pulmonary artery pressures
Pulmonary function testing	To measure lung volumes. Methacholine provocation challenge may identify airway hyperreactivity
Arterial blood gas	To provide information about altered pH, hypercapnia, hypocapnia, or hypoxemia

Creatine phosphokinase and troponin	If ischemia or infarction are suspected
TSH	If thyroid abnormality is suspected as a cause of dyspnea
Digoxin level	For patients taking digoxin
Treadmill stress test, stress thallium, or stress echocardiogram	For patients with known or suspected coronary artery disease in whom dyspnea may represent an anginal equivalent
Neck radiographs	If stridor is present or upper airway obstruction is suspected
D-dimer	If deep venous thrombosis or pulmonary embolism is suspected
Bilateral venous compression ultrasonography plus either ventilation–perfusion scan or pulmonary CT angiography, or pulmonary angiography	If pulmonary embolism is suspected
High-resolution computed tomography	May be helpful in diagnosing interstitial lung disease, pulmonary fibrosis, bronchiectasis, and pulmonary embolism
Holter monitor	To help diagnose intermittent arrhythmias that may result in dyspnea
Brain natriuretic peptide	May be useful in the diagnosis of heart failure
Cardiac catheterization	May be required to confirm or diagnose less common causes of pulmonary hypertension
Esophageal pH monitoring	To help establish gastroesophageal reflux as the cause of dyspnea

| Cardiopulmonary exercise testing | Helps quantify cardiac function, pulmonary gas exchange, ventilation, and physical fitness. May be useful in cases in which no apparent cause for dyspnea is found after a thorough evaluation |
| Lung biopsy | May be indicated if interstitial lung disease or malignancy are suspected |

Further reading

American Thoracic Society. Dyspnea: mechanisms, assessment, and management: a consensus statement. American Journal of Respiratory Critical Care Medicine 1999;159: 321–340.

Karnani NG, Reisfield GM, Wilson GR. Evaluation of chronic dyspnea. American Family Physician 2005;71: 1529–1537.

Mahler DA, Fierro-Carrion G, Baird JC. Evaluation of dyspnea in the elderly. Clinics in Geriatric Medicine 2003;19: 19–33.

Morgan WC, Hodge HL. Diagnostic evaluation of dyspnea. American Family Physician 1998; 57: 711–716.

Shiber JR, Santana J. Dyspnea. Medical Clinics of North America 2006;90: 453–479.

Zoorob RJ, Campbell JS. Acute dyspnea in the office. American Family Physician 2003;68: 1803–1810.

20 DYSURIA

General Discussion

Dysuria is the sensation of burning, pain, or discomfort on urination, most often the result of infection or inflammation of the bladder and/or urethra. Infection may present as urethritis, cystitis, prostatitis, or pyelonephritis. Although dysuria often is equated with urinary tract infection, dysuria also may result from vaginitis, malformations of the urinary tract, malignancy, hormonal conditions, trauma, interstitial cystitis, neurogenic conditions, and psychogenic disorders.

The timing of the dysuria may help predict the location of the problem in the urinary tract. Discomfort at the start of urination suggests a urethral source of inflammation, while pain occurring over the suprapubic area upon completion of urination often indicates inflammation of the bladder.

Dysuria is much more common in women than in men, and it affects older men more than younger men, reflecting the impact of benign prostatic hyperplasia (BPH).

Medications and Supplements Associated with Dysuria

Cantharidin

Cyclophosphamide

Dopamine

Penicillin G

Pumpkin seeds

Saw palmetto

Ticarcillin

Causes of Dysuria

Anatomic issues

- BPH
- Bladder diverticula
- Urethral stricture

Infection

- Cervicitis
- Cystitis
- Epididymo-orchitis
- Prostatitis
- Urethritis
- Vulvovaginitis

Hormonal causes

- Atrophy and dryness in postmenopausal women

Inflammatory disorders

- Autoimmune disorders
- Behçet's syndrome
- Reiter's syndrome

Medication and supplement side effects

Neoplasm

- Bladder cancer
- Penile cancer
- Prostate cancer
- Renal cell tumor
- Vaginal cancer
- Vulvar malignancy

Psychogenic disorders

- Anxiety
- Chemical dependency
- Chronic pain syndromes
- Depression
- Somatization
- Stress

Trauma

- Urethral instrumentation or catheter placement
- Urethral trauma during intercourse

Other causes

- Bicycle riding
- Horseback riding
- Interstitial cystitis
- Sensitivity to creams, sprays, soaps, or toilet paper
- Stones (renal, ureteral, and bladder)
- Urethral syndrome

Key Historical Features

✓ Onset and duration of dysuria

✓ Fever, chills, nausea, or vomiting

✓ Timing of dysuria, particularly if related to menstrual cycle

✓ Frequency of dysuria

✓   Severity

✓   Location of discomfort

✓   External vs internal dysuria

✓   Pain at onset of urination vs suprapubic pain after voiding

✓   Presence of hematuria

✓   Urinary frequency, urgency, or hesitation

✓   Nocturia

✓   Sexual habits

✓   Penile discharge

✓   Scrotal pain

✓   Perineal pain

✓   Vaginal discharge

✓   Dyspareunia

✓   Use of topical irritants such as lubricants, douches, or soaps

✓   Back pain

✓   Joint pain

✓   Ocular symptoms

✓   Oral mucosal symptoms

✓   Past medical history

✓   Past surgical history

✓   Sexual history, including history of sexually transmitted diseases

✓   Tobacco use

✓   Medications

✓   Family history

Key Physical Findings

✓   Fever

✓   Head and neck exam for conjunctivitis or oral ulcers

✓   Abdominal examination to assess the kidneys and bladder

✓   Back examination for costovertebral angle tenderness

✓   Pelvic examination in women

✓   Perineal, penile, and testicular examination in men

✓   Digital rectal examination

✓   Inguinal lymphadenopathy

✓   Extremity examination for joint swelling or tenderness

✓   Skin examination for rash

Suggested Work-Up

Urinalysis	To evaluate for pyuria or hematuria
Urine culture	To accurately diagnose infection and determine antimicrobial susceptibility of infecting bacteria
Vaginal wet-mount preparation	To detect *Trichomonas vaginalis* and *Candida* species
Urethral smear or urine ligase chain reaction and polymerase chain reaction tests for *Neisseria gonorrhoeae* and *Chlamydia trachomatis*	To detect *Neisseria gonorrhoeae* and *Chlamydia trachomatis* infections

Additional Work-Up

Urine cytology	If urinary tract malignancy is suspected
Cystoscopy	To detect bladder or urethral pathology and confirm the diagnosis of interstitial cystitis. Used in the evaluation of noninfectious hematuria
Renal ultrasonography	If kidney or ureter pathology such as abscess or hydronephrosis is suspected
Bladder ultrasonography	If bladder or urethral stones are suspected or if bladder diverticula are suspected
Plain films of kidneys, ureters, and bladder	For rapid evaluation of suspected renal stones

Contrast CT scan	To visualize avascular structure such as infarcts, (preferred) cysts, abscesses, and necrotic tumors
Noncontrast CT scan	To evaluate for renal stones/calcifications and to evaluate solid tissue in the urinary tract
Voiding cystourethrogram	To assess for abnormalities such as vesicoureteral reflux, neurogenic bladder, urethral strictures, diverticula, and BPH
Intravenous pyelography	To evaluate recurrent urinary tract infection or localize ureteral calculi
MRI with gadolinium enhancement	To identify urinary obstruction or mass in patients with renal insufficiency or allergy to iodinated contrast media

Further reading

Bremnor JD, Sadovsky R. Evaluation of dysuria in adults. American Family Physician 2002;65: 1589–1596.

Roberts RG, Hartlaub PP. Evaluation of dysuria in men. American Family Physician 1999; 60: 865–872.

Thomas A, Woodard C, Rovner ES, et al. Urologic complications of nonurologic medications. Urologic Clinics of North America 2003;30: 123–131.

21 | ERECTILE DYSFUNCTION

General Discussion

Erectile dysfunction is the inability to achieve or maintain a penile erection sufficient for satisfactory sexual performance. Erectile dysfunction may be divided into either psychogenic or organic origin. Current evidence suggests that up to 80% of cases have an organic cause. Of the organic causes, vasculogenic etiologies represent the largest group, though neurogenic and hormonal etiologies also are frequently implicated.

The evaluation of the patient with erectile dysfunction begins with a thorough history to assess the patient's sexual problems and to differentiate erectile dysfunction from other sexual problems such as a decreased libido or ejaculatory problems. The nature of the erectile dysfunction should be detailed, such as onset, duration, progression, the quality of erections, the presence or absence of nocturnal erections, and the presence or absence of dysfunction with masturbation. Past medical history and medication use are important historical features. Important elements of the social history include cigarette use, alcohol abuse, illicit drug use, relationship problems, and life stressors.

Medications Associated with Erectile Dysfunction

Alpha blockers

Anti-psychotics

Benzodiazepines

Beta blockers

Carbamazepine

Clonidine

Digoxin

Fibrates

Histamine H2 receptor blockers

Lithium

Ketoconazole

Methyldopa

Methotrexate

Metoclopramide

Monoamine oxidase inhibitors

Omeprazole

Opioids

Phenobarbital

Phenytoin

Reserpine

Selective serotonin reuptake inhibitors

Spironolactone

Statin medications

Thiazide diuretics

Tricyclic antidepressants

Causes of Erectile Dysfunction

Addison's disease

Aging

Alcohol abuse

Anatomic abnormalities

Anxiety

Atherosclerosis

Cavernosal disorders

COPD

Chronic renal failure

Cigarette smoking

Cushing's syndrome

Depression

Diabetes mellitus

Heart disease

Herniated disc

Hyperlipidemia

Hyperprolactinemia

Hypertension

Hyperthyroidism

Hypogonadism

Hypothyroidism

Ischemic heart disease

Lipid disorders

Liver disease

Marijuana use

Medications

Multiple sclerosis

Narcotic use

Pelvic radiation

Pelvic surgery

Pelvic trauma

Peripheral neuropathy

Peripheral vascular disease

Peyronie's disease

Renal failure

Social stressors

Spinal cord injury

Spinal disc herniation

Trauma

Vascular disease

Venous incompetence

Key Physical Findings

✓   Cardiovascular exam

- Blood pressure and pulse
- Signs of hypertensive or ischemic heart disease
- Abdominal or femoral artery bruits
- Peripheral pulses
- Skin and hair patterns suggestive of peripheral vascular disease

✓   Neurologic exam

- Signs of anxiety or depression
- Anal sphincter tone and anal reflex

✓   Genitourinary systems

- Phimosis or hypospadias
- Testicular size and other evidence of hypogonadism
- Evidence of Peyronie's disease
- Prostate gland for size, symmetry, and nodules

Suggested Work-Up

CBC	To evaluate for infection or polycythemia
Urinalysis	To screen for renal disease or urinary tract infection
BUN and creatinine	To evaluate for renal disease
Fasting lipid panel	To evaluate for lipid disorders

Fasting blood sugar	To evaluate for diabetes mellitus
TSH	To evaluate for thyroid disorders
Serum testosterone	To evaluate for low testosterone
Serum prolactin	To evaluate for hyperprolactinemia

Additional Work-Up

LH and FSH	In men with low testosterone to differentiate testicular from hypothalamic–pituitary dysfunction
MRI of the brain (pituitary)	In men with elevated prolactin level to rule out pituitary tumor

Further reading

Fazio L, Brock G. Erectile dysfunction: management update. Canadian Medical Association Journal 2004;170: 1429–1437.

Miller TA. Diagnostic evaluation of erectile dysfunction. American Family Physician 2000; 61: 95–104.

NIH Consensus Conference on Impotence. Journal of the American Medical Association 1993;270: 83–90.

Seftel AD, Mohammed MA, Althof SE. Erectile dysfunction: etiology, evaluation, and treatment options. Medical Clinics of North America 2004;88: 387–416.

Thomas DR. Medications and sexual function. Clinics in Geriatric Medicine 2003;19: 553–562.

22 FATIGUE

General Discussion

Fatigue is defined as a subjective state of sustained lack of energy or exhaustion with a decreased capacity for physical and mental work which persists despite sufficient rest. Fatigue is one of the most common complaints in adults presenting for primary care in the United States and must be differentiated from weakness or exertional difficulties.

Acute viral syndromes are a common cause of fatigue and usually are self-limited. Fatigue that persists longer than one month generally warrants investigation. Although fatigue usually is the symptom of which the patient complains, a careful history often will reveal associated symptoms. A targeted physical examination may lead to additional diagnostic clues. A laboratory examination may not be required in all cases of fatigue, but targeted testing may help the clinician reveal the cause of the patient's symptoms.

Depression is the most common cause of clinically important fatigue in patients presenting for primary care. Fatigue is common in the elderly population and may represent part of the normal aging process. However, fatigue should not be attributed to advanced age alone. Rather, fatigue as a consequence of advanced age should be a diagnosis of exclusion.

Medications Associated with Fatigue

Almost every medication may cause fatigue and should be considered in the evaluation of the patient with fatigue. The following categories of medications are more common causes of fatigue.

Antihistamines

Benzodiazepines

Beta blockers

Blood pressure medications

Diuretics

Glucocorticoids

Narcotic pain medications

NSAIDs

Selective serotonin reuptake inhibitors

Sleeping medications

Tricyclic antidepressants

Causes of Fatigue

Addison's disease

Advancing age

Alcohol abuse

Allergic rhinitis

Amebiasis

Anemia

Anorexia nervosa

Bipolar disorder

Blastomycosis

Bulimia nervosa

Cancer

Carbon monoxide poisoning

Chemotherapy

COPD

Chronic sinusitis

Coccidiomycosis

Cushing's disease

Cytomegalovirus infection

Dementia

Depression

Dermatomyositis

Diabetes

Domestic abuse

Drug abuse

Endocarditis

Epstein–Barr virus syndrome

Fibromyalgia

Giardiasis

Heart failure

Heavy metal exposure

Helminth infestation

Hepatitis B or C

Histoplasmosis

Hypercalcemia

Hyperthyroidism

Hypothyroidism

Liver disease

Lyme disease

Lymphoma

Malnutrition

Medications

Mixed connective tissue disease

Multiple sclerosis

Myasthenia gravis

Obesity

Occult malignancy

Parkinson's disease

Parvovirus B19 infection

Polymyalgia rheumatica

Polymyositis

Radiation therapy

Rheumatoid arthritis

Sarcoidosis

Significant weight loss

Situational stress

Sjögren's syndrome

Sleep apnea

Systemic lupus erythematosus

Temporal arteritis

Toxin exposure

Tuberculosis

Uremia

Viral infections

Key Historical Features

✓ Onset

✓ Nature of the fatigue

✓ Past medical history, including psychiatric history

✓ Medications

✓ Family history

✓ Social history

   • Travel

   • Alcohol use

   • Drug use

   • Dietary habits

- • Caffeine consumption
- • Life events/stressors, relationships with family members
✓ Review of systems
  - • Fever, chills
  - • Night sweats
  - • Weight loss or weight gain
  - • Appetite
  - • Arthralgias
  - • Myalgias
  - • Headache
  - • Adenopathy
  - • Paresthesias
  - • Sore throat
  - • Rash
  - • Sleep disturbance
  - • Anhedonia
  - • Weakness
  - • Problems with memory or concentration

Key Physical Findings

✓ Age

✓ Gender

✓ Weight

✓ Vital signs

✓ Head and neck examination for signs of anemia, sinusitis, oral ulcerations, postnasal drip, thyromegaly, or lymphadenopathy

✓ Ophthalmologic examination for signs of increased intracranial pressure, retinopathy, or anemia

✓ Cardiovascular examination, including jugular venous distension

✓ Pulmonary examination

✓ Abdominal examination for abdominal masses, hepatomegaly, splenomegaly, or ascites

✓ Examination of the musculature for signs of weakness or muscle atrophy

✓ Skin examination for color changes, rash, skin texture changes, or hair changes

✓   Genital examination

✓   Rectal examination, including stool guaiac

✓   Neurologic examination

Suggested Work-Up

Serial weight measurement	To help evaluate for depression or systemic illness
Monitoring of temperature	To help evaluate for infection or malignancy
CBC	To evaluate for infection or malignancy
Electrolytes	To evaluate for adrenal insufficiency
BUN and creatinine	To evaluate for renal failure
Glucose	To evaluate for diabetes mellitus
ALT and AST	To evaluate for hepatocellular disease
Total bilirubin	To evaluate for hepatitis or hemolysis
Albumin	To evaluate for malnutrition and hepatic synthetic dysfunction
Alkaline phosphatase	To evaluate for obstructive liver disease
Creatine kinase	To evaluate for muscle disease
Calcium	To help detect hyperparathyroidism, cancer, and sarcoidosis
Phosphorus	To evaluate for hypo- or hyperphosphatemia
ESR	To help detect collagen–vascular disease, malignancy, endocarditis, abscess, osteomyelitis, tuberculosis, etc.
TSH	To evaluate for hyper- and hypothyroidism
Urinalysis	To evaluate for proteinuria and renal disease

Additional Work-Up

Lyme serologies	If Lyme disease is suspected
HIV	If the patient is at risk for HIV infection
ANA	If lupus or other collagen vascular diseases are suspected
Hepatitis B and C screening	If the patient is at risk of hepatitis B or C or if the patient has abnormal liver function tests
Purified protein derivative (PPD) skin test	If the patient is at risk for tuberculosis or if tuberculosis is suspected clinically
Chest X-ray	If cardiopulmonary disease is suspected
Brucella titers	If brucellosis is suspected clinically
Monospot or Epstein–Barr titers	If mononucleosis/Epstein–Barr infection is suspected
Cytomegalovirus (CMV) titers	If CMV infection is suspected
Blood cultures	If endocarditis or bacteremia is suspected
Histoplasma antigen	If histoplasmosis is suspected
Adrenocorticotropic hormone (ACTH) test	If Cushing's disease is suspected
Tensilon test	If myasthenia gravis is suspected
Echocardiogram	If heart failure is suspected
Parvovirus IgM	If parvovirus infection is suspected
24-hour urine for heavy metals	If heavy metal exposure is suspected
Serum angiotensin converting enzyme (ACE) level	If sarcoidosis is suspected

Further reading

Cho WK, Stollerman GH. Chronic fatigue syndrome. Hospital Practice (Off Ed)
    1992:27: 221–224.

Craig T, Kakumanu S. Chronic fatigue syndrome: evaluation and treatment. American Family
    Physician 2002;65: 1083–1090.

Manzullo EF, Escalante CP. Research into fatigue. Hematology/Oncology Clinics of North
    America 2002;16: 619–628.

Morrison RE, Keating HJ. Fatigue in primary care. Obstetrics and Gynecology Clinics 2001;
    28: 225–240.

General Discussion

Fever of unknown origin (FUO) is defined as a temperature elevation of 101°F (38.3 °C) or higher for 3 weeks or longer, the cause of which is not diagnosed after 1 week of intensive in-hospital investigation. Some attempts have been made to change the definition of FUO in special populations, such as "classic FUO," "nosocomial FUO," "FUO in neutropenic patients," and "FUO in HIV patients." Although such categorization has its merits, the pathogens in each of these categories merely reflect the frequency distribution of diseases causing prolonged fevers in these categories. Such categorization does not significantly alter or improve the diagnostic approach.

Recent series show that the diseases responsible for FUO involve over 100 disorders. The differential diagnosis of FUO can be divided into four subgroups: infections, malignancies, autoimmune conditions, and miscellaneous. Traditionally, infectious diseases represent the largest group of illnesses causing FUOs. However, the incidence of malignancy responsible for FUO has increased and in some published series is the most common cause of FUOs. As the duration of the fever increases, the likelihood of an infectious etiology decreases.

Abdominal abscesses, tuberculosis, and endocarditis are the most common infectious causes of FUO. Hodgkin's and non-Hodgkin's lymphoma are the most common neoplastic diseases responsible for FUO. Adult Still's disease and temporal arteritis are the most common autoimmune causes of FUO.

Atypical presentation of infection is common in older adults, particularly the very old (80+ years). Normal body temperature and the amplitude of circadian rhythm are reduced in frail elderly individuals, but not necessarily in healthy older persons. Twenty to thirty percent of elderly individuals with serious infections present with an absent or blunted fever response. Connective tissue diseases are identified as the cause of the illness with a relatively high frequency in patients older than 65 years. This is primarily because temporal arteritis and polymyalgia rheumatica are common in this age group.

Fever may be the sole or the most prominent feature of an adverse drug reaction.

Rash or eosinophilia may occur, though neither is common. Drug fever is a diagnosis of exclusion and may be confirmed by withdrawal of the offending medication.

Historical clues and physical findings, if present, provide the most useful diagnostic information in the evaluation of FUO. Repeated re-questioning and re-examination over time is extremely important as findings that were not initially apparent may become so and provide important clues to the diagnosis. Testing should be guided by the history and physical examination. It is not cost effective to order batteries of screening tests without some clinical suspicion for a diagnosis. The diagnostic objective is to use the history, physical examination, and laboratory data to establish a pattern of organ involvement.

Between 7 and 30% of FUO cases remain undiagnosed after thorough evaluation. However, fever resolves in the majority of these patients within a short time, and the mortality rate is 3% 5 years later. Only rarely did a serious disorder emerge later.

Medications Associated with FUO

Allopurinol

Aminoglycosides

Amphotericin

Atropine

Captopril

Cephalosporins

Cimetidine

Clindamycin

Clofibrate

Erythromycin

Heparin

Hydralazine

Hydrochlorothiazide

Interferon

Interleukin-2

Isoniazid

Macrolides

Meperidine

Methyldopa

Nifedipine

Nitrofurantoin

Penicillins

Phenytoin

Procainamide

Quinidine

Rifampin

Sulfonamides

Vancomycin

Causes of FUO

Infections

- Abdominal abscesses
- Amebiasis
- Blastomycosis
- Brucellosis
- Cat-scratch disease
- Coccidioidomycosis
- Colorado tick fever
- Complicated urinary tract infection
- Cytomegalovirus mononucleosis
- Dengue
- Dental abscesses
- Encephalitis
- Endocarditis
- Epstein–Barr virus
- Filariasis
- Histoplasmosis
- Human immunodeficiency virus
- Leptospirosis
- Lyme disease
- Lymphocytic choriomeningitis
- Malaria
- Meningitis (chronic)
- *Mycobacterium avium–intracellulare* complex
- Osteomyelitis
- Pelvic abscesses
- *Pneumocystis carinii* pneumonia
- Prostatitis
- Relapsing fever
- Salmonella
- Septic arthritis
- Sinusitis
- Syphilis
- Tuberculosis (especially extrapulmonary)
- Tularemia
- Typhoid fever
- Visceral leishmaniasis

Malignancies

- Angio-immunoblastic lymphadenopathy with dysproteinemia
- Atrial myxoma
- CNS malignancies
- Chronic leukemia
- Colorectal carcinoma
- Hepatoma
- Lymphoma (Hodgkin's and non-Hodgkin's)
- Malignant histiocytosis
- Metastatic disease
- Multiple myeloma and other myelodysplastic syndromes
- Pancreatic carcinoma
- Pheochromocytoma
- Renal cell carcinoma
- Sarcomas

Autoimmune conditions

- Adult Still's disease
- Behcet's syndrome
- Crohn's disease
- Cryoglobulinemia
- Familial Mediterranean fever
- Inflammatory bowel disease
- POEMS syndrome
- Polyarteritis nodosa
- Polymyalgia rheumatica
- Reiter syndrome
- Rheumatoid arthritis
- Rheumatoid fever
- Sjögren's syndrome
- Systemic lupus erythematosus
- Temporal arteritis
- Vasculitides
- Wegener's granulomatosis

Miscellaneous

- Allergic alveolitis
- Aortic dissection
- Cirrhosis (especially alcoholic)
- Deep venous thrombosis

- Drug-induced fever
- Erythema multiforme
- Factitious fever
- Hematoma
- Hepatitis
- Hypergammaglobulinemia IgD syndrome
- Kikuchi's disease (histocytic necrotizing adenitis)
- Pancreatitis
- Pulmonary embolism
- Retroperitoneal fibrosis
- Sarcoidosis
- Schnitzler syndrome
- Serum sickness
- Subacute thyroiditis
- Sweet's syndrome
- Thrombophlebitis
- Thrombotic thrombocytopenic purpura
- Tumor necrosis factor receptor-associated periodic syndrome
- Vitamin B_{12} deficiency

Key Historical Features

✓ Fever pattern

✓ Recent contact with persons exhibiting similar symptoms

✓ Arthralgias

✓ Rash

✓ Sore throat

✓ Past medical history

✓ Past surgical history

✓ Family history

✓ Medications

✓ Recent travel

✓ Work environment

✓ Exposure to pets and other animals

✓ Alcohol use

✓ Smoking history

✓ Intravenous drug use

Key Physical Findings

✓   Vital signs

✓   General physical appearance

✓   Head and neck examination for evidence of sinusitis, evidence of temporal arteritis, oropharyngeal lesions or ulcerations, tender teeth, lymphadenopathy, or eye findings

✓   Thyroid examination for enlargement or tenderness

✓   Cardiac examination for murmurs

✓   Pulmonary examination

✓   Abdominal examination for hepatic abnormalities, splenomegaly, or adenopathy

✓   Skin and nail examination for skin lesions, petechiae, splinter hemorrhages, subcutaneous nodules, or clubbing

✓   Lower extremity examination for evidence of deep venous tenderness

✓   Genital examination for testicular or epididymal nodules

✓   Rectal examination for perirectal fluctuance or tenderness. Prostate examination for prostatic tenderness or fluctuance

Suggested Work-Up

CBC	To evaluate for infection or hematologic abnormalities
ESR	To evaluate for evidence of inflammation
Electrolytes	To evaluate for metabolic abnormalities
Serum transaminases and alkaline phosphatase	To evaluate for liver disease
Urinalysis	To evaluate for urinary tract infection or other urinary abnormalities
Urine culture	To evaluate for urinary tract infection
Blood cultures	To evaluate for endocarditis and to identify blood-borne infections
Serum protein electrophoresis	To evaluate for multiple myeloma

PPD skin test	To evaluate for tuberculosis
Chest radiograph	To screen for infection, collagen vascular disease, or malignancy

Additional Work-Up

CT of abdomen/pelvis with contrast	To evaluate for abscess or malignancy Should be considered early in the diagnostic process
Lower extremity venous compression ultrasound	To evaluate for deep venous thrombosis
Urine and sputum cultures for acid fast bacilli (AFB)	If pulmonary or extrapulmonary tuberculosis is suspected
VDRL	To evaluate for syphilis
HIV test	To evaluate for HIV infection
Serology for CMV, EBV, ASO titer	If CMV, EBV, or Streptococcal disease is suspected
Sinus radiographs or CT	If sinusitis is suspected
Echocardiogram (transthoracic or transesophageal)	If bacterial endocarditis is suspected
Lumbar puncture	If CNS infection, malignancy, or autoimmune disease is suspected
Rheumatoid factor and ANA	If autoimmune conditions are suspected
Temporal artery biopsy	If temporal arteritis is suspected
Chest CT with contrast	If nonhematologic malignancy is suspected
Mammography	To evaluate for breast cancer
Stool guaiac	To evaluate for gastrointestinal blood loss

Upper/lower endoscopy	If gastrointestinal malignancy is suspected
Bone scan	If nonhematologic malignancy, metastatic disease, or osteomyelitis is suspected
Radionuclide scanning (gallium 67, technetium Tc 99m, or indium-labeled leukocytes)	To detect inflammatory conditions and neoplastic lesions that may be underdiagnosed by CT scans. Gallium 67 scan is best for infection and malignancy. Indium-labeled leukocytes may help diagnose occult septicemia. Technetium Tc 99m may help diagnose acute infection and inflammation of bones and soft tissue
Bone marrow biopsy	If hematologic malignancy is suspected
Biopsy of suspicious lymph nodes	To help evaluate for malignancy or infectious cause
Biopsy of suspicious skin lesions	To obtain histologic clues to the diagnosis

Further reading

Armstrong W, Kazanjian P. Fever of unknown origin in the general population and in HIV-infected persons. In: Cohen J, Powderly WG, eds. Infectious diseases, 2nd ed. Edinburgh: Mosby, 2004.

Carsons SE. Fever in rheumatic and autoimmune disease. Infectious Disease Clinics of North America 1996;10: 67–84.

Cunha BA. Fever of unknown origin (FUO). In: Gorbach SL, Bartlett JB, Blacklow NR, eds. Infectious diseases, 2nd ed. Philadelphia: WB Saunders; 1996.

Cunha BA. Fever of unknown origin. Infectious Disease Clinics of North America 1996; 10: 111–127.

Mackowiak PA, Durack DT. Fever of unknown origin. In: Mandell GL, Bennett JE, Dolin R, eds. Principles and practice of infectious diseases, 6th ed. New York: Churchill Livingstone; 2005.

Norman DC, Yoshikawa TT. Fever in the elderly. Infectious Disease Clinics of North America 1996;10: 93–99.

Roth AR, Basello GM. Approach to the adult patient with fever of unknown origin. American Family Physician 2003;68: 2223–2228.

24 FIBROMYALGIA

General Discussion

The 1990 American College of Rheumatology classification criteria for fibromyalgia has two components: (1) the presence of widespread pain for more than 3 months and (2) the presence of 11 tender points among 18 specified sites as outlined below. Estimates of prevalence are 3.4% for women and 0.5% for men.

The diagnosis of fibromyalgia can be made largely by pattern recognition. Fibromyalgia is a common clinical pain disorder in which the physical finding of palpable fibromyalgia tender points (FTPs) is associated with characteristic symptoms of generalized muscular aching, fatigue, stiffness, and nonrestorative sleep. Over three-quarters of individuals with fibromyalgia have these characteristic symptoms. Less common features that generally occur in 25–50% of cases of fibromyalgia include headache, irritable bowel syndrome, psychological distress, Raynaud's phenomenon, subjective swelling, nondermatomal paresthesia, and marked functional disability. Other somatic complaints include palpitations, dyspareunia/pelvic pain, temporomandibular pain, chronic rhinitis or "allergies," and cognitive difficulties such as memory impairment or concentration issues.

The somatic complaints distinguish fibromyalgia from rheumatoid arthritis (RA). However, fibromyalgia frequently coexists with other rheumatic diseases, especially systemic lupus erythematosus and RA. The differential diagnosis of fibromyalgia includes hypothyroidism, arthritis, polymyalgia rheumatica, osteomalacia, myofascial pain syndrome, metabolic and inflammatory myopathies, spondyloarthropathy, radiculopathy, and cardiac or pleuritic pain. The major challenge for the clinician is to distinguish fibromyalgia from an inflammatory or metabolic myopathy.

Muscular aching and stiffness in fibromyalgia are more proximal than distal, although the patient may complain of hurting all over. Palpation of an FTP causes pain localized to the area of palpation, and the pain does not radiate to adjacent areas and no pain is experienced at sites proximal or distal to the examining finger. No muscle induration is palpable.

Medications Associated with Myalgias

Clofibrate

Colchicine

Danazol

Gemfibrozil

Glucocorticoids

Hydralazine

Hydroxychloroquine

Lovastatin

Penicillamine

Phenytoin

Procainamide

Rifampin

Sulfonamides

Valproic acid

Vincristine

Zidovudine

Selected Causes of Myalgias

Amyotrophic lateral sclerosis

Collagen vascular disease

Dermatomyositis

Diabetes mellitus

Drug-induced myopathic syndromes

- Alcohol
- Cocaine
- Heroin
- Ipecac
- L-tryptophan
- Medications listed above

Familial periodic paralysis

Fibromyalgia

Guillain–Barré syndrome

Hyperthyroidism

Hypothyroidism

Inclusion body myositis

Infectious myositis (bacterial, viral, fungal, parasitic)

Myasthenia gravis

Occult or metastatic carcinoma

Polymyalgia rheumatica

Polymyositis

Porphyria

Temporal arteritis

Key Historical Features

- ✓ Chronicity of pain
- ✓ Intensity of pain
- ✓ Nature of pain
- ✓ Location(s) of pain
- ✓ Triggering factors
- ✓ Aggravating factors
- ✓ Presence of fatigue
- ✓ Presence of stiffness
- ✓ Sensation of joint swelling
- ✓ Presence of poor sleep or nonrestorative sleep
- ✓ Headache
- ✓ Cognitive difficulties
- ✓ Auditory/vestibular/ocular complaints
- ✓ Symptoms of irritable bowel syndrome
- ✓ Palpitations
- ✓ Dyspareunia
- ✓ Temporomandibular pain
- ✓ Other constitutional symptoms
- ✓ Mental stress, coping skills
- ✓ Quality of life
- ✓ Physical functioning and activities
- ✓ Perceived disability
- ✓ Past medical history
- ✓ Psychiatric history
- ✓ Past surgical history
- ✓ Medications
- ✓ Family medical history
- ✓ Use of alcohol, tobacco or drugs
- ✓ Current employment status
- ✓ Review of systems
- ✓ History of abuse

Key Physical Findings

The most important physical examination for a diagnosis of fibromyalgia is to systematically palpate the 18 sites suggested by the American College of Rheumatology criteria shown in the figure:

- Bilateral occiput (at the suboccipital muscle insertion)
- * Bilateral low cervical (at the anterior aspect of the intertransverse spaces between C5 and C7)
- Bilateral trapezius (mid-point of the upper border)
- Bilateral supraspinatus (origin of this muscle above the scapular spine near the border)
- Bilateral second rib (just lateral to the costochondral junctions on upper surface)
- Bilateral lateral epicondyle (2 cm distal to the epicondyle)
- Bilateral gluteal (at the upper outer quadrant of the buttock)
- Bilateral greater trochanter (posterior to the trochanter)
- Bilateral knee (medial fat pad proximal to the joint line)

Additional items in the physical exam include:

✓ Vital signs

✓ General appearance

✓ Affect

✓ Head and neck exam for dry mouth or evidence of temporomandibular joint dysfunction

✓ Examination of the thyroid gland

✓ Examination for lymphadenopathy

✓ Abdominal examination

✓ Examination of the extremities for joint swelling or other evidence of connective tissue disease

✓ Neurologic examination for cranial nerves, reflexes, muscle strength, sensory functions, and cerebellar signs

Suggested Work-Up

Laboratory or radiologic testing is not necessary for making a diagnosis of fibromyalgia. The tests outlined below are generally recommended to rule out other underlying disorders. Routine testing for rheumatoid factor or ANA is not recommended.

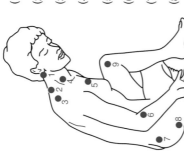

(1) insertion of nuchal muscles into occiput;

(2) upper border of trapezius-mid-portion;

(3) muscle attachments to upper medial border of scapula;

(4) anterior aspects of the C5, C7 intertransverse spaces;

(5) 2nd rib space - about 3 cm lateral to the sternal border;

(6) muscle attachments to lateral epicondyle;

(7) upper outer quadrant of gluteal muscles;

(8) muscle attachments just posterior to greater trochanter;

(9) medial fat pad of knee proximal to joint line.

A total of eleven or more tender points in conjunction with a history of widespread pain is characteristic of the fibromyalgia syndrome.

Figure 24-1. The American College of Rheumatology Criteria Recommended Tender point Locations. Locations of 18 (9 pairs) tender points as recommended in the American College of Rheumatology 1990 Criteria. From Bennett RM, Kelly WN, Harris ED, Ruddy S, Sledge CB (eds). Textbook of Rheumatology, Philadelphia: WB Saunders Co; 1997:511–519.

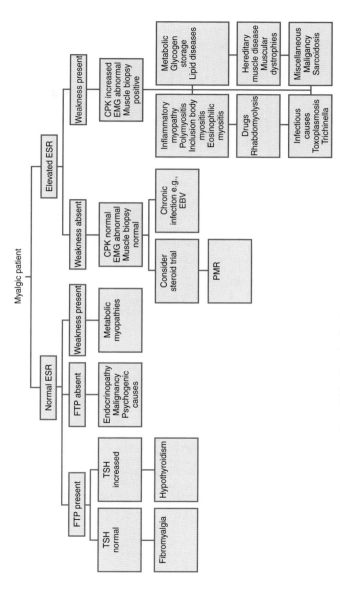

Figure 24-2. Algorithm for the investigation of the myalgic patient.

ESR	An elevated ESR makes fibromyalgia an unlikely primary diagnosis
TSH	To evaluate for hypothyroidism
CBC	To evaluate for anemia or cytopenia
Electrolytes, BUN, creatinine	To evaluate for underlying metabolic disorders and monitoring for medication side effects
AST and ALT	To evaluate for hepatic dysfunction
Serum calcium	To evaluate for hypo- or hypercalcemia

The following figure provides an algorithmic approach to the evaluation of the myalgic patient. The physical examination should concentrate on determining whether true muscle weakness is present and whether a high tender point count can be demonstrated. Patients can then be divided into two groups depending upon whether the ESR is elevated.

Additional Work-Up

X-rays of the spine	May be considered for middle-aged and elderly patients to evaluate for pathologic changes in the spine
Sleep study	May be considered if the history suggests a primary sleep disorder such as sleep apnea, REM sleep behavioral disorder, periodic limb movement disorder, or narcolepsy

Further reading

McCain GA. A cost-effective approach to the diagnosis and treatment of fibromyalgia. Rheumatic Diseases Clinics of North America 1996;22: 323–349.

Millea PJ, Holloway RL. Treating fibromyalgia. American Family Physician 2000;62: 1575–1582.

Winfield JB. Pain in fibromyalgia. Rheumatic Diseases Clinics of North America 1999; 25: 55–79.

Yunus MB. A comprehensive medical evaluation of patients with fibromyalgia syndrome. Rheumatic Diseases Clinics of North America 2002;28: 201–217.

General Discussion

Galactorrhea is the inappropriate production of milk from the breast in the absence of pregnancy or beyond 6–12 months postpartum in a nonbreastfeeding woman. The discharge of milk may be unilateral or bilateral, may be intermittent or persistent, and may vary in terms of volume. Galactorrhea may also occur in males and in infants and teenage girls.

Distinguishing galactorrhea from other forms of nipple discharge usually is straightforward. The discharge in galactorrhea has the appearance of milk, occurs from multiple ducts in the nipple, most commonly occurs bilaterally, and usually is spontaneous.

When nipple discharge is consistent with galactorrhea, the medical history often will reveal the etiology. Important elements of the history and physical exam are outlined below.

Medications Associated with Galactorrhea

Amphetamines

Butyrophenones

Calcium channel blockers

Cimetidine

Codeine

Methyldopa

Metoclopramide

Morphine

Oral contraceptives

Phenothiazines

Prochlorperazine

Reserpine

Risperidone

Selective serotonin reuptake inhibitors

Tricyclic antidepressants

Causes of Galactorrhea

Bronchogenic carcinoma

Chronic renal failure

Estrogen withdrawal

Heroin use

Hypothalamic lesions

- Craniopharyngioma
- Empty sella syndrome
- Pituitary stalk lesions
- Primary hypothalamic tumor
- Sarcoidosis
- Tuberculosis

Hypothyroidism

Idiopathic

Medications

Neonatal galactorrhea

Neurogenic causes

- Breast stimulation
- Burns
- Chest surgery
- Shingles

Pituitary tumors (usually prolactinoma)

Thoracic neoplasms

Key Historical Features

✓ Duration of galactorrhea

✓ Unilateral or bilateral

✓ Associated breast mass

✓ Medications

✓ Medical history, particularly thyroid disorders or renal failure

✓ Surgical history, especially recent chest surgery is important

✓ Family history, especially thyroid disorders or multiple endocrine neoplasia increases the risk for these processes

✓ Reproductive history

- Oral contraceptives are the most common medication-related cause of galactorrhea
- Oligomenorrhea, amenorrhea, infertility, decreased libido, or impotence suggest hyperprolactinemia
- Amenorrhea may indicate pregnancy or pituitary tumor

✓ Constitutional symptoms

- Fatigue and cold intolerance suggest hypothyroidism
- Nervousness, heat intolerance, unusual sweating, and weight loss despite a normal or increased appetite suggest thyrotoxicosis

- • Polyuria and polydipsia suggest pituitary or hypothalamic disease
✓ Skin symptoms

  - • Dry skin suggests hypothyroidism
  - • Acne and hirsutism suggest hyperandrogenism
✓ Gastrointestinal symptoms

  - • Constipation suggests hypothyroidism
✓ Neurologic symptoms

  - • Headache, visual disturbance, and seizure suggest pituitary or hypothalamic disease

Key Physical Findings

✓ Vital signs

✓ Poor growth or short stature suggestive of hypothyroidism, hypopituitarism, or chronic renal failure

✓ Acromegaly or gigantism suggestive of pituitary tumor

✓ Breast examination for nodules and discharge and determine whether the discharge is from one duct or multiple

✓ Cardiac examination

  - • Bradycardia suggests hypothyroidism
  - • Tachycardia suggests thyrotoxicosis
✓ Skin examination for dry skin, coarse hair, and myxedema suggesting hypothyroidism or hirsutism and acne suggesting hyperandrogenism

✓ Head and neck examination for goiter suggesting hypothyroidism

✓ Eye examination for visual field defect or papilledema suggesting pituitary tumor or intracranial mass

✓ Neurologic examination for hand tremor suggesting thyrotoxicosis or a cranial neuropathy suggesting pituitary tumor or intracranial mass

Suggested Work-Up

The evaluation of galactorrhea should proceed in a stepwise fashion and be guided by findings from the history and physical examination.

Pregnancy test	To evaluate for pregnancy in women of childbearing age
Serum prolactin	To evaluate for pituitary adenoma
TSH	To evaluate for hypo- or hyperthyroidism

Additional Work-Up

If hyperprolactinemia is confirmed, medications that may cause elevated prolactin levels should be withheld if possible. The prolactin level should then be repeated.

If true hyperprolactinemia is found, MRI with gadolinium enhancement should be performed to evaluate the pituitary fossa. A serum prolactin level greater than 200 ng/mL is strongly suggestive of pituitary adenoma.

FSH, LH, DHEAS	To evaluate for hyperandrogenism when it is suggested by history and physical examination
BUN and creatinine	When chronic renal failure is suggested by history and physical examination
MRI of brain with gadolinium	When intracranial mass is suggested by history and physical examination

Further reading

Benjamin F. Normal lactation and galactorrhea. Clinical Obstetrics and Gynecology 1994; 37: 887–897.

Falkenberry SS. Nipple discharge. Obstetrics and Gynecology Clinics 2002;29: 21–29.

Jardines L. Management of nipple discharge. The American Surgeon 1996;62: 119–122.

Leung, AKC, Pacaud D. Diagnosis and management of galactorrhea. American Family Physician 2004;70: 543–550.

Luciano AA. Clinical presentation of hyperprolactinemia. Journal of Reproductive Medicine 1999;44(12 suppl): 1085–1090.

Serri O, Chik CL, Ur E, et al. Diagnosis and management of hyperprolactinemia. Canadian Medical Association Journal 2003;169: 575–581.

Spack NP, Neinstein LS. Galactorrhea. In: Neinstein LS, ed. Adolescent health care: a practical guide, 4th ed. Philadelphia: Lippincott Williams & Wilkins; 2002:1045–1051.

General Discussion

Gynecomastia, the excessive development of the male mammary glands, which occurs when there is a disturbance in the normal ratio of circulating androgens to estrogens. The prevalence of gynecomastia is estimated to be approximately 40% and usually presents bilaterally. There is a progressive increase in the prevalence of gynecomastia with advancing age.

The central issue is to distinguish true gynecomastia from fatty enlargement of the breasts (lipomatosa). When this distinction is in doubt after careful physical examination, mammography or ultrasonography may be performed.

It is important to remember that an underlying diagnosis is made in less than half of patients referred for gynecomastia. As such, not all cases of gynecomastia require extensive evaluation. Indications for further work-up include a negative medication and drug history, breast tenderness, or a mass larger than 4 cm in diameter.

Medications Associated with Gynecomastia

Amiodarone

Anabolic steroids

Angiotensin-converting enzyme (ACE) inhibitors

Calcium-channel blockers

Chemotherapy agents

- Alkylating agents
- Busulfan
- Imatinib
- Nitrosoureas
- Vincristine

Cimetidine

Cisplatin

Clomiphene

Diazepam

Diethylstilbestrol

Digoxin

Efavirenz

Estrogens

Ethionamide

Etomidate

Finasteride

Flutamide

Furosemide

Gonadotropins

Growth hormone

Haloperidol

Isoniazid

Ketoconazole

Melatonin

Methadone

Methotrexate

Methyldopa

Metoclopramide

Metronidazole

Omeprazole

Paroxetine

Penicillamine

Phenothiazines

Phenytoin

Progesterones

Ranitidine

Reserpine

Risperidone

Spironolactone

Sulindac

Theophylline

Tricyclic antidepressants

Causes of Gynecomastia

Adrenal disease

Alcohol abuse

Amphetamine use

Chronic renal failure

Congenital defects

- Androgen resistance
- Anorchia

- Defects of testosterone synthesis
- Klinefelter syndrome

Hermaphroditism

Heroin use

HIV infection

Hyperthyroidism

Idiopathic

Increased estrogen production

Liver disease

Malnutrition

Marijuana use

Medications

Testicular failure

- Castration
- Granulomatous disease
- Neurologic disease
- Trauma
- Viral orchitis

Testicular tumors

Thyrotoxicosis

Key Historical Features

✓   Age

✓   Onset

✓   Rate of growth

✓   Pain/tenderness

✓   Past medical history

✓   Medications

✓   Drug history

Key Physical Findings

✓   Fatty tissue vs true gynecomastia

✓   Examination of the testes

✓   Evidence of systemic disease such as thyrotoxicosis, liver disease, or adrenal disease

Suggested Work-Up

AST, ALT, gamma-glutamyl transpeptidase (GGT), total bilirubin	To evaluate liver function
TSH	To evaluate for hyperthyroidism
Serum prolactin	To evaluate for prolactinoma
Serum androstenedione	To evaluate for feminizing adrenal states
Plasma estradiol	To evaluate for congenital adrenal hyperplasia and feminizing adrenal tumors
Plasma human chorionic gonadotropin (hCG)	To evaluate for testicular tumor and retroperitoneal histologic unmixed seminoma
Plasma luteinizing hormone and testosterone	To evaluate for testicular failure, Sertoli cell tumor, androgen resistance, and gonadotropin-secreting tumor

Additional Work-Up

Mammogram or ultrasound	If breast malignancy is suspected
Chromosomal karyotype	If both testes are small
Testicular ultrasound	If the testes are asymmetric, to evaluate for testicular tumor

Further reading

Wilson JD. Endocrine disorders of the breast. In: Isselbacher KJ, Braunwald E, Wilson JD, eds. Harrisons's textbook of internal medicine, 13th ed. New York: McGraw-Hill; 1994: 2037–2039.

Wise GJ, Roorda AK, Kalter R. Male breast disease. Journal of the American College of Surgeons 2005;200: 255–269.

General Discussion

Hair loss, or alopecia, can be classified in various ways, but the most common classification distinguishes nonscarring from scarring alopecia. The hair loss of scarring alopecia is permanent while nonscarring alopecia usually is reversible. When a patient presents with hair loss, it is important to determine if he or she is experiencing hair shedding, which is significant amounts of hair coming out, or hair thinning, which is more visible scalp without noticeable amounts of hair falling out.

Every hair follicle goes through three phases: anagen (growth), catagen (transition between growth and resting), and telogen (resting). At any given time, approximately 85% of scalp follicles are in the anagen phase, and follicles remain in this phase for an average of 3 years. The catagen phase affects 2–3% of hair follicles at a time. The telogen phase occurs last, during which 10–15% of hair follicles undergo a rest period for about 3 months. At the end of telogen, the dead hair is ejected from the skin and the cycle is repeated.

Alopecia areata is patchy hair loss of autoimmune origin. It usually occurs in well-circumscribed patches, but also may involve the entire scalp (alopecia totalis) or body (alopecia universalis). The involved scalp may be normal or show subtle erythema or edema. Short hairs that taper as they approach the scalp surface, known as exclamation-mark hairs, are characteristic of alopecia areata. Alopecia areata may be associated with thyroid disease, vitiligo, or atopy.

Androgenic alopecia, the most common form of alopecia in men and women, is also known as male-pattern balding, female-pattern balding, and common balding. Most patients with androgenic alopecia complain of thinning hair rather than shedding of hair. In some women, androgenic alopecia may be a manifestation of hyperandrogenism, so the history should focus on related signs such as menstrual irregularities, infertility, hirsutism, and acne. In an otherwise healthy woman with slowly progressive androgenic alopecia and no signs or symptoms of hyperandrogenism, no laboratory testing is required. Men with androgenic alopecia do not require a laboratory evaluation.

Cicatricial alopecia results from a condition that damages the scalp and hair follicle. Examination typically reveals plaques of erythema with or without scaling. Syphilis, tuberculosis, AIDS, herpes zoster, discoid lupus erythematosus, sarcoidosis, radiation therapy, and scalp trauma such as burns have been associated with cicatricial alopecia. If the cause of the disorder is not apparent, a punch biopsy of the scalp may be helpful in making the diagnosis.

Scarring alopecia represents a heterogeneous group of diseases manifested by erythematous papules, pustules, or scaling centered around hair follicles, resulting in eventual obliteration of follicular orifices.

Senescent (senile) alopecia is the steady decrease in the density of scalp hair which occurs in all persons as they age. Patients will note a slow, steady, diffuse pattern of thinning hair beginning about age 50 years.

Syphilitic alopecia should be considered in every patient with unexplained hair loss. Hair loss may be rapid or slow and insidious and may be patchy (moth-eaten in appearance) or diffuse. Syphilic alopecia is a noninflammatory, nonscarring alopecia without erythema, scaling, or induration. However, in symptomatic syphilic alopecia, the patchy or diffuse alopecia is associated with the papulosquamous lesions of secondary syphilis on the scalp or elsewhere.

Telogen effluvium occurs when an abnormally high percentage of normal hairs from all areas of the scalp enter telogen, the resting phase of hair growth. Many factors can precipitate telogen effluvium, especially stress. This disorder also may develop because of normal physiologic events such as the postpartum state or because of medications or endocrinopathies. Telogen effluvium usually begins 2–6 months after the causative event and lasts for several months. Hair loss is diffuse and may also affect pubic and axillary hair. Telogen effluvium is noninflammatory, and the scalp surface appears normal. The hair pull test is positive, though the telogen count usually does not exceed 50%.

Tinea capitis is a common condition caused by dermatophytes. Tinea capitis presents with one or several patches of alopecia as well as scalp inflammation. Broken-off hair shafts may create a black dot appearance on the scalp. Fungal organisms can be displayed in a KOH preparation or may be cultured after adequate scraping of hair stubs from the periphery of the lesion.

Traction alopecia is a form of traumatic alopecia associated with certain methods of hair styling including braiding, tight curlers, and ponytails. The outermost hairs are subjected to the most tension, and a zone of alopecia develops between braids and along the margin of the scalp.

Trichotillomania is a psychiatric impulse-control disorder in which the patient plucks the hairs. The pattern of hair loss often suggests the diagnosis. One or more well-circumscribed areas of hair loss may be present, often in a bizarre pattern with incomplete areas of clearing. The scalp may be normal or may show areas of erythema or pustule formation. Laboratory testing is not required, though psychiatric consultation may be considered.

Medications Associated with Hair Loss

Anticonvulsants

Antithyroid agents

Chemotherapy agents

Etretinate

Heparin

Hormones

Causes of Hair Loss

Alopecia areata

Androgenic alopecia

Scarring (cicatricial) alopecia

- AIDS
- Discoid lupus erythematosus of the scalp
- Dissecting cellulitis
- Folliculitis decalvans
- Herpes zoster
- Lichen planopilaris
- Pseudopelade
- Radiation therapy
- Sarcoidosis
- Scalp trauma (burns, injuries)
- Syphilis
- Tuberculosis

Senescent (senile) alopecia

Syphilitic alopecia

Telogen effluvium

- Drugs
- Early stages of androgenetic alopecia
- Heavy metals
- High fever
- Hypothyroidism
- Major surgery
- Medications
- Physiologic effluvium of the newborn
- Postpartum effluvium
- Severe chronic illness
- Severe diets (crash or liquid protein diets)
- Severe infection
- Severe psychological stress

Tinea capitis

Traction alopecia

Traumatic alopecia and cosmetic alopecia

Trichotillomania

Key Historical Features

✓ Shedding vs thinning

✓ Duration of the problem

✓ Whether hair is broken or shed at the roots

✓ Grooming practices (chemical treatments such as relaxers, bleaching, coloring, or blow drying on high heat)

✓ Diet

✓ Physical or emotional stressors within the previous 3–6 months

✓ Medical history

✓ Medications

✓ Family history of hair loss, including maternal relatives, paternal relatives, siblings, and children

✓ Menstrual irregularities, infertility, hirsutism, or acne in women suspected of having hyperandrogenism

Key Physical Findings

✓ Pattern of hair loss (patterned vs diffuse hair loss)

✓ Examination of the scalp for erythema, scaling, pustules, edema, bogginess, sinus tract formation, or obliteration of follicular openings

✓ Examination of the hair shaft for caliber, shape, length, and fragility

✓ Thyroid examination

✓ Pubic or axillary hair loss

✓ Evidence of hirsutism

Suggested Work-Up

Hair pull test — 50–60 hairs are grasped between the thumb and the index and middle fingers, then the hairs are gently but firmly pulled. A negative test is six or fewer hairs obtained. A positive test is more than six hairs obtained and indicates a process of active hair shedding. Microscopic evaluation of the hairs may be performed. The hair pull test is helpful in suspected cases of telogen effluvium, tinea capitis, systemic diseases, alopecia areata, alopecia totalis, alopecia universalis, and environmental factors.

| Serologic test for syphilis | Recommended for all patients with unexplained hair loss to rule out syphilis |

Additional Work-Up

| KOH prep for fungal elements or fungal culture of skin | In patchy forms of alopecia to rule out fungal infection |

| Total testosterone, free testosterone, dehydroepiandrosterone sulfate, and prolactin level | In women suspected of having hyperandrogenism |

| TSH, RPR, prolactin, CBC, chemistry profile, ESR, ANA, rheumatoid factor, and hair pluck test for telogen:anagen ratio | In patients with telogen effluvium |

| CBC, ESR, ANA, rheumatoid factor | In patients with alopecia areata |

| KOH examination or culture swab | In suspected cases of tinea capitis |

| Scalp biopsy | If the etiology is unclear or if the patient fails to improve after appropriate treatment |

Further reading

Sperling LC, Mezebish DS. Hair diseases. Medical Clinics of North America 1998; 82: 1155–1169.

Springer K, Brown M, Stulberg DL. Common hair loss disorders. American Family Physician 2003;68: 93–102.

Thiedke CC. Alopecia in women. American Family Physician 2003;67: 1007–1014.

28 HEADACHE

General Discussion

The majority of patients with headache experience either migraine, tension-type, or medication rebound headaches. Serious or anatomical causes of headaches are uncommon but have to be considered when a patient presents with a headache. Headaches, and migraines in particular, occur more frequently in women and can be very disabling.

Migraine headaches are usually unilateral, throbbing, and worsen with exercise and typically last 4–72 hours. They are often associated with nausea, vomiting, and sensitivity to light and sound. Associated auras are usually visual or sensory disturbances. Most severe, recurrent headaches are migraines.

Tension headaches, on the other hand, are usually mild and frequently can be treated with over-the-counter pain medications. Unlike migraines, they are usually bilateral and not affected by physical activity. They are often described as a pressure, ache, tightness, or "band-like constriction" around the head. Location of symptoms is commonly cervical, occipital, or temporal, though numerous variants exist. Nausea with or without vomiting may be associated with tension headaches.

Medication rebound headache should be high on the differential diagnosis for any patient with chronic daily headaches. A patient may begin with migraine or tension-type headache on an episodic basis, but then transform to medication rebound headache with the frequent use of analgesics. Medication rebound headache may be caused by either over-the-counter or prescription medications. Combination medications such as Excedrin (caffeine, aspirin, and acetaminophen) are often implicated.

Less common types of headaches include trigeminal neuralgia and idiopathic intracranial hypertension (also known as pseudotumor cerebri or benign intracranial hypertension). Trigeminal neuralgia occurs in the distribution of the trigeminal nerve, lasts only seconds to minutes, and feels like electric shocks. Headaches caused by trigeminal neuralgia can be triggered by touching the affected area. Idiopathic intracranial hypertension (IIH) is associated with papilledema and visual changes and can lead to blindness. Young obese women are at particular risk for IIH.

When evaluating a patient with a headache it is essential to rule out a serious cause of headache by assessing any red flags during the history and physical. These red flags include neurologic symptoms or signs, older age at onset, systemic illness or symptoms (such as fever, cancer, pregnancy or postpartum status, use of anticoagulants), sudden onset, new headache, different or progressive headache, headache awakening the patient from sleep, and occipital headache. Headaches that can have severe consequences if they remain undiagnosed include subarachnoid hemorrhage (sudden onset) and other intracranial bleeds, IIH, meningitis (associated with fever, neck rigidity) and other infections, brain neoplasm (may be associated with seizures), and giant cell arteritis (associated with temporal artery tenderness, diminished temporal artery pulse, jaw claudication, polymyalgia rheumatica, and visual changes).

Potential indicators of intracranial pathology in patients with sudden-onset acute headache are occiptonuchal location, age greater than 40 years, and an abnormal neurologic examination. Symptoms of particular concern in patients with non-acute headache include increasing frequency or progressive symptoms, neurologic signs or symptoms, or headache awakening the patient from sleep (not explained by cluster headache or typical migraine).

Medications Associated with Headache

Cimetidine

Dextroamphetamine

Diclofenac

Dipyridamole

Estrogen

Famotidine

Griseofulvin

Hydralazine

Isosorbide

Lansoprazole

Levodopa

Methylphenidate

Minoxidil

Monosodium glutamate

Nalidixic acid

Niacin

Nifedipine

Nitrites

Nitroglycerin

Omeprazole

Phenothiazines

Piroxicam

Progesterone

Pseudoephedrine

Ranitidine

Reserpine

SSRIs

Sulfates

Sulfonamides

Tamoxifen

Tetracyclines

Theophyllines

Trimethoprim

Tyramine

Vitamin A

Causes/Types of Headache

Acute angle-closure glaucoma

Arteriovenous malformation

Brain abscess

Brain tumor

Carbon monoxide exposure

Carotid artery dissection

Cerebral venous thrombosis

Cervical spondylosis

Chronic paroxysmal hemicrania

Cluster headache

Coital headache

Encephalitis

Exercise headache

Generalized seizure

Giant cell arteritis (temporal arteritis)

Granulomatous angiitis

HIV infection

Hydrocephalus

Hypercapnia due to chronic obstructive lung disease

Hypertensive encephalopathy

Hyperthyroidism

Hypothyroidism

IIH

Intracerebral hemorrhage

Ischemic stroke

Medication rebound headache

Meningitis

Migraine headache

Polyarteritis nodosa (vasculitis)

Preeclampsia

Postepidural headache

Posttraumatic headache

Rheumatoid arthritis (vasculitis)

Sinusitis

Sleep apnea

Subarachnoid hemorrhage

Systemic lupus erythematosus (vasculitis)

Temporomandibular joint (TMJ) syndrome

Tension headache

Trigeminal neuralgia

Key Historical Features

✓   Location of headache

✓   Nature of headache

✓   Pattern of headache

✓   Duration of headache

✓   Frequency of headache

✓   Severity of headache

✓   Age when headaches first experienced

✓   Triggers (exercise, food, sex, coughing, cold liquids)

✓   Associated symptoms

- Fever
- Nausea or vomiting
- Stiff neck
- Neck pain
- Vision changes
- Rash
- Nasal congestion
- Facial pain
- Jaw claudication
- Myalgias

✓   Auras

✓   Recent lumbar puncture/epidural injection

- ✓ Recent trauma
- ✓ Past medical history, especially:
  - Prior headaches
  - Cancer
  - Lung disease
  - HIV infection
  - Thyroid disease
  - Hypertension
  - Stroke
  - Preeclampsia
  - Heart disease
- ✓ Past surgical history
- ✓ Obstetrical history
- ✓ Social history
  - Tobacco, alcohol, drugs, caffeine use
  - Diet and physical activity
  - Domestic violence
- ✓ Family history, especially of headaches
- ✓ Medications, including anticoagulants, pain medications
- ✓ Neurologic symptoms
  - Change in mental status
  - Memory loss
  - Personality changes
  - Numbness
  - Weakness
  - Balance problems
  - Speech difficulty
  - Loss of consciousness
  - Dizziness
  - Tinnitus
  - Seizures
- ✓ Psychological symptoms
  - Stressors
  - Sleep history and whether headaches awaken patient from sleep
  - History or symptoms of depression, anxiety, or personality disorders

✓   Gynecologic/obstetric symptoms

  •   Relation of headache to menstrual cycle

  •   Date of last menstrual period

✓   Gastrointestinal symptoms

  •   Right upper quadrant abdominal pain may be associated with preeclampsia

Key Physical Findings

✓   Vital signs, especially hypertension or fever

✓   Body mass index

✓   General assessment of well-being and mental status

✓   Head and neck examination for evidence of ear infection, sinusitis, TMJ syndrome, neck stiffness, neck tenderness, or temporal artery tenderness, swelling, or erythema

✓   Funduscopic examination to evaluate for papilledema

✓   Neurologic examination (complete)

✓   Musculoskeletal examination for any muscle tenderness or trigger points

Suggested Work-Up

In the absence of neurologic findings, episodic migraine does not require imaging studies. The evidence is less clear for chronic migraine and chronic nonmigraine headaches. The American Academy of Neurology states that neuroimaging should be considered in patients with unexplained abnormal findings on the neurologic examination, but states that there is no clear evidence to recommend MRI or CT as the initial examination.

Patients who have had a stable headache pattern for at least 6 months rarely have significant intracranial pathology. In the absence of worrisome features, these patients do not require imaging.

Features that raise the index of suspicion for a pathologic cause in patients with chronic or recurrent headaches include systemic symptoms or illness (especially fever, change in mentation, anticoagulation, current or recent pregnancy, or cancer), neurologic symptoms or signs (papilledema, asymmetric cranial nerve or motor function, or abnormal cerebellar function), recent or sudden onset of headache, onset after 40 years of age, or a previous headache history that is different, or progression of headaches.

MRI of brain or CT of brain	If there are features that raise the index of suspicion for a pathologic cause, as outlined above.

Additional Work-Up

Complete blood count	If infection or anemia is suspected
HIV test	If the patient is at risk for HIV infection
Lumbar puncture	If meningitis or subarachnoid hemorrhage is suspected
Blood culture	If meningitis is suspected
ESR	If giant cell arteritis is suspected
Temporal artery biopsy	If giant cell arteritis is suspected
TSH	If thyroid disease is suspected
Urine pregnancy test	If pregnancy is suspected
Urinalysis	To evaluate for proteinuria in a pregnant patient
Liver function tests, creatinine, uric acid, lactate dehydrogenase	If preeclampsia is suspected
PT, PTT, international normalized ratio (INR)	If preeclampsia or hemorrhage is suspected or a patient is taking an anticoagulant
Sinus X-rays or CT	If sinusitis is suspected

Further reading

Dodick DW. Clinical clues and clinical rules: primary vs secondary headache. Advances in the Study of Medicine 2003;3: S550–S555.

Frishberg BM. The utility of neuroimaging in the evaluation of headache in patients with normal neurologic examinations. Neurology 1994;44: 1191–1197.

Johnson CJ. Headache in women. Primary Care: Clinics in Office Practice 2004;31: 417–428.

Levin M. The many causes of headache: migraine, vascular, drug-induced, and more. Postgraduate Medicine 2002;112(6): 67–68, 71–72, 75–76.

Maizels M. The patient with daily headaches. American Family Physician 2004;70: 2299–2306.

Marcus DA. Focus on primary care: diagnosis and management of headache in women. Obstetrical and Gynecological Survey 1999;54(6): 395–402.

Paulson GW. Headaches in women, including women who are pregnant. American Journal of Obstetrics and Gynecology 1995;173(6): 1734–1741.

Silberstein SD. Practice parameter: evidence-based guidelines for migraine headache (an evidence-based review): report of the Quality Standards Subcommittee of the American Academy of Neurology. Neurology 2000;55: 754–762.

29 HEARING LOSS

General Discussion

More than 28 million Americans have some degree of hearing impairment, and 25–40% of those aged 65 years or older are hearing impaired. The differential diagnosis of hearing loss can be simplified by determining whether the hearing loss is conductive or sensorineural. Conductive hearing loss is caused by imperfect function of the external canal, tympanic membrane, or ossicles, which are located in the outer and middle ear. Sensorineural hearing loss is caused by injury to the cochlea or auditory nerve in the inner ear. A mixed hearing loss may also occur which involves both conductive and sensorineural loss.

More than 90% of hearing loss is sensorineural. Presbycusis, sensorineural loss related to aging, is the most common cause of hearing loss in the United States. This type of hearing loss is typically gradual, bilateral, and characterized by high-frequency hearing loss.

The physician may be faced with a patient with sudden hearing loss. The etiology of sudden sensorineural hearing loss is not yet clear, though a variety of mechanisms such as viral infections, microcirculatory injuries, and immune-mediated disorders have been proposed. A viral infection of the cochlea is believed to be the most common cause of sudden sensorineural hearing loss.

Menière's disease is characterized by the tetrad of unilateral fluctuating hearing loss, a sensation of aural fullness, tinnitus, and vertigo. Sudden, low-frequency hearing loss is a hallmark of Menière's disease, though higher frequencies are affected as the disease progresses. Hearing loss is typically associated with episodic and recurrent paroxysms of vertigo.

The evaluation of hearing loss begins with a thorough history and physical examination followed by audiography. The goal of the audiologic evaluation is to determine the laterality, severity, and site of lesion of hearing loss. Patients with asymmetric sensorineural hearing loss require MRI of the brain with gadolinium to rule out acoustic neuroma and other cerebellopontine-angle tumors.

Medications Associated with Hearing Loss

Aminoglycosides
Chemotherapeutics agents
- Carboplatin
- Cisplatin
- Vincristine sulfate

Diuretics
- Ethacrynic acid
- Furosemide

Erythromycin

Quinine

Salicylates (especially aspirin)

Vancomycin

Causes of Hearing Loss

Conductive hearing loss

- Cerumen impaction
- Cholesteatoma
- Cyst
- Exostoses
- Foreign bodies
- Glomus tumor
- Middle ear effusion
- Osteomas
- Otitis externa
- Otosclerosis
- Tumor (adenoma, carcinoma, fibroma, melanoma, papilloma, sarcoma)
- Tympanic membrane perforation
- Tympanosclerosis

Sensorineural hearing loss

Bilateral hearing loss

- Autoimmune processes
- Noise trauma
- Ototoxin exposure
- Presbycusis

Unilateral hearing loss

- Acoustic neuroma
- Menière's disease
- Perilymph fistula
- Temporal bone fracture
- Vascular occlusive disease
- Viral cochleitis

Key Historical Features

✓ Onset of hearing loss

✓ Progression of hearing loss (sudden or gradual)

✓   Involvement of one or both ears

✓   Dizziness or vertigo

✓   Tinnitus

✓   Sensation of aural fullness

✓   Ear or head trauma

✓   Ear discharge

✓   Ear pain

✓   Past medical history, especially history of ear infections or ear injury.
    Also note history of atherosclerotic disease

✓   Medications

✓   Family history of hearing loss

✓   Exposure to loud noises

✓   Tobacco use

Key Physical Findings

✓   Visualization and palpation of the auricle and periauricular
    tissues

✓   Otoscopic examination of the external auditory canal for cerumen,
    foreign bodies, and abnormalities of the canal skin. The mobility, color,
    and surface anatomy of the tympanic membrane should be noted.
    A pneumatic bulb may be used to assess the tympanic membrane
    and the aeration of the middle ear

✓   Weber test

✓   Rinne test

✓   Head and neck examination

✓   Cranial nerve examination

Suggested Work-Up

Audiography	To determine the laterality, severity, and site of lesion of hearing loss
MRI of the brain with gadolinium enhancement	For patients with asymmetric sensorineural hearing loss to rule out acoustic neuroma and other cerebellopontine-angle tumors

Additional Work-Up

Serum IgE, ESR, ANA, anticardiolipin antibody, and circulating anti-neutrophil cytoplasmic antibody (C-ANCA)	If an autoimmune process is suspected

Further reading

Isaacson JE, Vora NM. Differential diagnosis and treatment of hearing loss. American Family Physician 2003;68: 1125–1132.

Jerger J, Chmiel R, Wilson N, et al. Hearing impairment in older adults: new concepts. Journal of the American Geriatrics Society 1995;43: 928–935.

Marcincuk MC, Roland PS. Geriatric hearing loss: understanding the causes and providing appropriate treatment. Geriatrics 2002;57: 44–59.

Palmer CV, Ortmann A. Hearing loss and hearing aids. Neurologic Clinics 2005;23: 901–918.

Yueh B, Shapiro N, MacLean CH, et al. Screening and management of adult hearing loss in primary care. Journal of the American Medical Association 2003;289:1976–1985.

30 HEMATOSPERMIA

General Discussion

Hematospermia, or blood in the ejaculate, may result from many different causes. Most men with hematospermia are young, with infections or inflammatory disorders accounting for 39% of cases. Malignancies and trauma each account for 2% of cases. Up to 46% of cases are labeled idiopathic, while a variety of other conditions account for the remaining cases.

For the majority of patients, no significant work-up is needed, but for a minority of patients, hematospermia may be a sign of serious urologic disease.

The history should focus on trauma and infection. The past medical history may play a role if there is a history of a bleeding disorder, hypertension, or previous malignancy. A sexual history should be included. Important elements of the physical exam are outlined below.

Causes of Hematospermia

Prostatic Sources

- Polyps
- Vascular lesions
- Calculi
- Inflammation
- Malignancy
- Bleeding following prostate biopsy

Bladder Sources

- Bladder tumor

Urethral Sources

- Urethritis
- Urethral cyst
- Urethral polyp
- Condylomata
- Urethral stricture

Seminal Vesicle Sources

- Seminal vesicle cyst
- Seminal vesicle malignancy

Infectious Sources

- Tuberculosis
- Schistosomiasis

- Cytomegalovirus
- Hydatid disease

Trauma

- Testicular injury
- Peyronie's disease
- Following hemorrhoidal injection
- Urethral instrumentation

Systemic Disorders

- Bleeding diatheses
- Hypertension
- Chronic liver disease
- Lymphoma

Other

- Seminal vesicular amyloidosis
- Seminal vesiculovenous fistula

Key Physical Findings

✓ Blood pressure

✓ Inspection of the penis

✓ Palpation of the vasa for swelling, induration, or nodularity

✓ Palpation of the testes

✓ Digital rectal examination of the prostate gland

Suggested Work-Up

Urinalysis and urine culture (preferably 72 hours after ejaculation)	To evaluate for hematuria
PSA	To evaluate for prostate cancer
Urethral swabs or urine evaluation for gonorrhea and chlamydia	To evaluate for gonococcal or chlamydial urethritis in younger men or those at risk
PPD	If the history suggests exposure to tuberculosis

Additional Work-Up

If the initial work-up demonstrates abnormalities or if the patient has persistent hematospermia after empiric treatment with antibiotics, urologic evaluation should be considered. Additional studies may include:

Transrectal ultrasound or cystourethroscopy	May help identify the possible etiology when it is not clear from initial work-up
MRI	May be helpful when seminal vesical or prostate hemorrhage is suspected

Further reading

Fletcher MS, Herzberg Z, Prior JR. The aetiology and investigation of hemospermia. British Journal of Urology 1981;53: 669–671.

Ganabathi K, Chadwick D, Feneley RC, et al. Hemospermia. British Journal of Urology 1992;69: 225–230.

Jones DJ. Hemospermia: a prospective study. British Journal of Urology 1991;67: 88–90.

Leary FJ, Aguilo JJ. Clinical significance of hemospermia. Mayo Clinic Proceedings 1974; 49: 815–817.

Mulhall JP, Albertsen PC. Hemospermia: diagnosis and management. Urology 1995; 46: 463–467.

Papp G, Molnar J. Causes and differential diagnosis of hematospermia. Andrologia 1981; 13: 474–478.

General Discussion

Definitions of microscopic hematuria vary from one to more than 10 red cells per high-power field. The American Urological Association has issued guidelines for the evaluation of microscopic hematuria in adults and defines clinically significant microscopic hematuria as three or more red blood cells per high-power field on microscopic evaluation of urinary sediment from two of three properly collected urinalysis specimens. However, each laboratory establishes its own thresholds based on the method of detection used.

Dipstick testing for heme lacks specificity, since the presence of myoglobin or hemoglobin may result in a positive test when the urine contains no red cells. If the dipstick test is positive, the presence of red cells should be confirmed by microscopic examination of the urine. If the urine dipstick reveals blood as well as leukocyte esterase, nitrites, and bacteria consistent with urinary tract infection, treatment with antibiotics is appropriate. If the hematuria resolves with treatment, no additional evaluation is necessary but serum creatinine should be measured.

Microscopic hematuria may be transient, caused by vigorous exercise, mild trauma, sexual intercourse, or by menstrual contamination. If transient microscopic hematuria is suspected, urinalysis should be repeated 48 hours after discontinuation of these activities. Persistent microscopic hematuria warrants further evaluation.

Causes of microscopic hematuria may be classified as either glomerular or nonglomerular in origin. IgA nephropathy is the most common glomerular cause. Nonglomerular causes involve the kidney and upper urinary tract and include nephrolithiasis, neoplasm, polycystic kidney disease, medullary sponge kidney, papillary necrosis, hypercalciuria, and hyperuricosuria. Causes involving the lower urinary tract include disorders of the bladder, urethra, and prostate such as bladder and prostate cancer.

The urinalysis is the most important test in the evaluation of hematuria because it often distinguishes glomerular from nonglomerular bleeding. If proteinuria is detected on dipstick testing, total urinary protein excretion should be quantified. Twenty-four-hour urinary protein excretion greater than 300 mg suggests the kidney as a source of microscopic hematuria. Other findings that support a glomerular etiology include renal insufficiency, red cell casts, or dysmorphic red blood cells. When glomerular bleeding is suggested, no urologic evaluation is necessary. Proteinuria or renal insufficiency with microscopic hematuria warrants referral to a nephrologist for evaluation and possible renal biopsy.

If a glomerular source is ruled out or considered unlikely, the upper urinary tract should be imaged. Excretory urography, ultrasonography,

CT, or MRI may be used. A CT scan without the use of contrast is appropriate as the first test for patients with suspected stone disease. When there is no clinical suspicion of stone disease, CT urography should be performed first without contrast and then with contrast. CT is more expensive than excretory urography and ultrasonography, but is the best imaging modality for the evaluation of urinary stones, renal and perirenal infections, and associated complications. In addition, excretory urography and ultrasonography often require additional imaging to further evaluate cysts. When CT is unavailable, excretory urography or ultrasound are reasonable alternatives individually or in combination. Ultrasonography is advised in place of CT for patients with renal failure, pregnancy, or hypersensitivity to contrast medium.

The source of microscopic hematuria is not found in about 70% of cases after urinalysis for evidence of glomerular hematuria and imaging of the upper urinary tract. The work-up usually proceeds with evaluation of the lower urinary tract. Cystoscopy is appropriate if risk factors for bladder cancer are present and in older men with asymptomatic microscopic hematuria. Cytologic analysis of voided urine is less sensitive than cystoscopy in the detection of bladder cancer, but has high specificity. The sensitivity is improved if specimens of urine are obtained from the first voiding in the morning on 3 consecutive days.

Patients at risk for significant disease include those with a smoking history; occupational exposure to benzenes or aromatic amines; age over 40 years; history of gross hematuria; history of urologic disease; history of irritative voiding symptoms; history of urinary tract infection; history of pelvic irradiation; or analgesic abuse.

A thorough evaluation of the urinary system may fail to identify a source of microscopic hematuria in 19–68% of patients. In patients with a negative initial evaluation of asymptomatic microscopic hematuria, consideration should be given to repeating urinalysis, voided urine cytology, and blood pressure determination at 6, 12, 24, and 36 months. Additional evaluation, including repeat imaging and cystoscopy, may be warranted in patients with persistent hematuria in whom there is a high index of suspicion for significant underlying disease. If gross hematuria, abnormal urinary cytology, or irritative voiding symptoms in the absence of infection develop, reevaluation should be undertaken immediately. This may include cystoscopy, urinary cytology, or repeat imaging.

Medications Associated with Hematuria

Aminoglycosides

Amitriptyline

Anticonvulsants

Aspirin

Busulfan

Captopril

Cephalosporins

Chlorpromazine

Ciprofloxacin

Cyclophosphamide

Diuretics

Furosemide

Heparin

Indinavir

Mirtazapine

Nonsteroidal anti-inflammatory drugs

Omeprazole

Oral contraceptives

Penicillins

Quinine

Rifampin

Ritonavir

Triamterene

Trimethoprim-sulfamethoxazole

Vincristine

Warfarin

Causes of Microscopic Hematuria

Glomerular causes

- IgA nephropathy
- Fabry's disease
- Goodpasture's syndrome
- Hemolytic uremic syndrome
- Henoch–Schönlein purpura
- Hereditary nephritis (Alport's syndrome)
- Lupus nephritis
- Membranoproliferative glomerulonephritis
- Mesangial proliferative glomerulonephritis
- Mild focal glomerulonephritis of other causes
- Nail–patella syndrome
- Polyarteritis
- Postinfectious glomerulonephritis (endocarditis or viral)

- Poststreptococcal glomerulonephritis
- Thin basement membrane disease
- Wegener's granulomatosis

Nonglomerular causes

- Upper urinary tract causes
  - Cytomegalovirus
  - Epstein–Barr virus
  - Hereditary nephritis
  - Hypercalciuria
  - Hyperuricosuria
  - Loin pain–hematuria syndrome
  - Lymphoma
  - Malignant hypertension
  - Medications
  - Medullary sponge kidney
  - Multicystic kidney disease
  - Nephrolithiasis
  - Papillary necrosis
  - Polycystic kidney disease
  - Pyelonephritis
  - Renal arteriovenous malformation
  - Renal cell carcinoma
  - Renal infarction
  - Renal venous thrombosis
  - Renal trauma
  - Renal tuberculosis
  - Sarcoidosis
  - Schistosomiasis
  - Sickle cell trait or disease
  - Sjögren's syndrome
  - Solitary renal cyst
  - Syphilis
  - Toxoplasmosis
  - Tuberculosis
  - Ureteral stricture
  - Ureteral transitional-cell carcinoma

- Lower urinary tract causes
  - Benign bladder polyps and tumors
  - Benign prostatic hypertrophy
  - Benign ureteral polyps and tumors
  - Bladder cancer
  - Calculi
  - Coagulopathy
  - Congenital abnormalities
  - Cystitis
  - Endometriosis
  - Epididymitis
  - Foreign bodies
  - Perineal irritation
  - Posterior ureteral valves
  - Prostate cancer
  - Prostatitis
  - Radiation-induced inflammation
  - Schistosomiasis
  - Transitional cell carcinoma of ureter or bladder
  - Trauma (catheterization, blunt trauma)
  - Urethral and meatal strictures
  - Urethritis

Other causes

- Benign hematuria
- Exercise hematuria
- Factitious hematuria
- Menstrual contamination
- Overanticoagulation with warfarin
- Sexual intercourse

Key Historical Features

✓ Irritative voiding

✓ Past medical history, especially urologic history or pelvic irradiation

✓ Medications

✓ Cigarette smoking

✓ Travel history

✓ Occupational exposure to benzene or aromatic amines

Key Physical Findings

✓   Vital signs, especially blood pressure measurement

✓   General examination

✓   Cardiac examination for irregular rhythm to suggest atrial fibrillation or new murmur to suggest endocarditis

✓   Abdominal examination for bruits, masses, organomegaly, or aortic aneurysm

✓   Back examination for costovertebral angle tenderness

✓   Genital examination

✓   Urethral and vaginal examination in women

✓   Prostate examination in men

✓   Extremity examination for peripheral edema or petechiae

Suggested Work-Up

Urinalysis	To evaluate for bacteriuria and pyuria
Urine culture	Should be obtained if the urinalysis reveals bacteriuria or pyuria
Serum creatinine	To evaluate for renal insufficiency
CT urography without and with contrast (excretory urography and ultrasonography are alternatives when CT is not available or is too expensive. Ultrasonography is advised in place of CT for patients with renal failure, pregnancy, or hypersensitivity to contrast medium	To evaluate the upper urinary tract for renal-cell carcinoma, transitional cell carcinomas, urolithiasis, cystic disease, and obstructive lesions
Cytologic analysis of urine (first void in the morning on 3 consecutive days)	To evaluate for bladder cancer and carcinoma in situ
Cystoscopy	Recommended for all persons with asymptomatic microscopic hematuria who are older than 40 years and those who are younger but have risk factors for bladder cancer

Patient with newly diagnosed asymptomatic microscopic hematuria*

Exclude benign causes, including menstruation, vigorous exercise, sexual activity, viral illness, trauma and infection

If one or more of the following are present:
Microscopic hematuria accompanied by significant proteinuria†
Dysmorphic red blood cells or red cell casts
Elevated serum creatinine level (based on normal reference ranges for men and women)

Evaluation for primary renal disease

If conditions suggestive of primary renal disease are not present (i.e., normal creatinine level, absence of proteinuria, absence of dysmorphic red blood cells or red cells casts), or if any of the following are present:
Smoking history
Occupational exposure to chemicals or dyes (benzenes or aromatic amines)
History of gross hematuria
Age>40 years
Previous urologic disorder or disease
History of irritative voiding symptoms
History of recurrent urinary tract infection despite appropriate use antibiotics

Urologic evaluation

*— The recommended definition of microscopic hematuria is three or more red blood cells per high-power field on microscopic evaluation of two of three properly collected specimens.

†— Proteinuria of 1+ or greater on dipstick urinalysis should prompt a 24-hour urine collection to quantitate the degree of proteinuria. A total protein excretion of >1000 mg per 24 hours (1 g per day) should prompt a thorough evaluation or nephrology referral. Such an evaluation should also be considered for lower levels of proteinuria (>500 mg per 24 hours [0.5 g per day]), particularly if the protein excretion is increasing or persistent, or if there are other factors suggestive of renal parenchymal disease.

Figure 31-1. Initial evaluation of newly diagnosed asymptomatic microscopic hematuria.

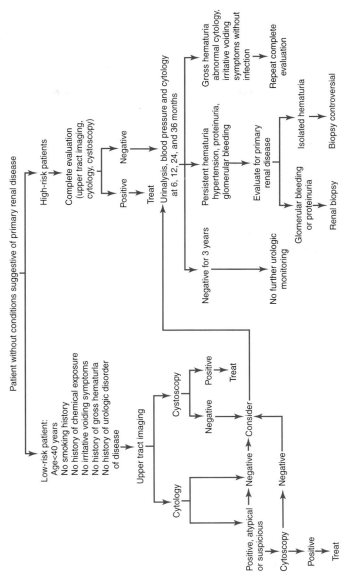

Figure 31-2. Urologic evaluation of asymptomatic microscopic hematuria.

Additional Work-Up

Urinary protein to urinary creatinine concentration ratio or 24-hour urine collection

If proteinuria is detected on dipstick testing to determine total protein excretion

Further reading

Ahmed Z, Lee J. Hematuria and proteinuria. Medical Clinics of North America 1997;
    81: 641–652.
Cohen RA, Brown RS. Microscopic hematuria. New England Journal of Medicine 2003;
    348: 2330–2338.
Feld LG, Waz WR, Perez LM, et al. Hematuria. An integrated medical and surgical approach.
    Pediatric Clinics of North America 1997;44: 1191–1210.
Grossfeld GD, Carroll PR. Evaluation of asymptomatic microscopic hematuria. Urologic Clinics
    of North America 1998;25: 661–676.
Grossfeld GD, Wolf JS, Litwin MS, et al. Asymptomatic microscopic hematuria in adults:
    summary of the AUA best practice policy recommendations. American Family Physician
    2001;63: 1145–1154.
Harper M, Arya M, Hamid R, et al. Haematuria: a streamlined approach to management.
    Hospital Medicine 2001;62: 696–698.
Mazhari R, Kimmel PL. Hematuria: an algorithmic approach to finding the cause. Cleveland
    Clinic Journal of Medicine 2002;69: 870–876.
McDonald MM, Swagerty D. Assessment of microscopic hematuria in adults. American Family
    Physician 2006;73: 1748–1754.
Sokolosky MC. Hematuria. Emergency Medicine Clinics of North America 2001;19: 621–632.
Thaller TR, Wang LP. Evaluation of asymptomatic microscopic hematuria in adults. American
    Family Physician 1999;60: 1143–1154.
Yun EJ, Meng MV, Carroll PR. Evaluation of the patient with hematuria. Medical Clinics
    of North America 2004;88: 329–343.

General Discussion

Hemoptysis, the coughing up of blood from the respiratory tract, must be differentiated from hematemesis (the vomiting of blood) and pseudohemoptysis (blood in the sputum that originates in the nasopharynx or oropharynx). Blood in the lungs may originate from bronchial arteries, pulmonary arteries, bronchial capillaries, and alveolar capillaries.

Tuberculosis is the most common cause of hemoptysis worldwide. However, bronchitis, bronchiectasis, and bronchogenic carcinoma represent the most common causes of hemoptysis in the United States, with acute and chronic bronchitis accounting for up to 50% of cases. The underlying cause is never found in 15% to 30% of cases of hemoptysis.

The appearance of the blood and the clinical history can offer clues to the cause of hemoptysis. Red, frothy blood mixed with purulent sputum usually is associated with an underlying pulmonary infection. Weight loss raises concern for cancer, especially in a smoker over the age of 40 years who has had hemoptysis lasting longer than 1 week. Night sweats, fever, and generalized illness may suggest tuberculosis as the cause. Persons with recent travel to Asia, South American, or the Middle East may present with hemoptysis as a result of parasitic infections such as schistosomiasis. A monthly pattern of bleeding in a menstruating woman suggests pulmonary endometriosis. Goodpasture's syndrome should be considered if the urinalysis reveals hematuria.

Medications Associated with Hemoptysis

Anticoagulants

Penicillamine

Causes of Hemoptysis

Anticoagulation therapy

Bioterrorism

- Pneumonic plague
- T2 mycotoxin
- Tularemia

Bronchiectasis

Coagulopathy

- Hemophilia
- von Willebrand's disease
- Thrombocytopenia

Cocaine use

Cystic fibrosis

Goodpasture's syndrome

Heart failure

Infection

- Ascariasis
- Bronchitis
- Fungal infections (aspergilloma)
- Hydatid cyst
- Lung abscess
- Mycobacteria, especially tuberculosis
- Necrotizing pneumonia
- Paragonimiasis
- Schistosomiasis

Lymphangioleiomyomatosis

Neoplasm

- Adenoma
- Bronchogenic carcinoma
- Metastatic lung cancer

Pulmonary endometriosis

Trauma

Vascular

- Arteriovenous malformation
- Broncho-arterial fistula
- Mitral stenosis
- Pulmonary embolism/infarct
- Rupture of pulmonary artery by balloon-tipped catheter
- Ruptured thoracic aneurysm

Vasculitis

- Behcet's disease
- Wegener's granulomatosis

Key Historical Features

✓ Color of blood

✓ Patterns of bleeding

✓ Quantity of blood loss

✓ Fever

✓   Weight loss

✓   Night sweats

✓   Generalized illness

✓   Chest pain

✓   Hematuria

✓   Changes in color of stool

✓   Association of hemoptysis with menstruation

✓   Past medical history (especially history of bleeding disorders)

✓   Family history

✓   History of smoking

✓   Recent travel

✓   Complete review of systems

Key Physical Findings

✓   Vital signs

✓   Pulse oximetry

✓   Inspection of the nose and oropharynx

✓   Evaluation for lymphadenopathy

✓   Cardiovascular exam (especially for congestive heart failure)

✓   Examination of the thorax for trauma or other abnormalities

✓   Pulmonary exam (auscultation for stridor, wheezing, crackles, or diminished breath sounds)

✓   Examination of the extremities for cyanosis, clubbing, or edema

Suggested Work-Up

Pulse oximetry	To evaluate oxygenation status
Chest X-rays	To evaluate for underlying pathology such as tumors, infiltrates, atelectasis, and cavitary lesions
CT scan with intravenous contrast enhancement	Useful in many cases of hemoptysis when chest X-ray is normal. Useful for diagnosing bronchiectasis, peripheral masses, alveolar consolidation, and abnormal enhancing vessels

Sputum for Gram stain and acid-fast stain. Sputum culture for bacteria, fungus, and mycobacterium	If an infectious etiology is suspected
Sputum smear for cytology	If cancer is suspected by history, if the patient is a smoker, if the patient is older than 40 years, or if the patient has suspicious findings on chest X-ray
CBC	To quantify blood loss, detect evidence of infection, or detect thrombocytopenia
Prothrombin time and partial thromboplastin time	To evaluate for coagulopathy

Additional Work-Up

Bronchoscopy	May be used to visualize the origin of bleeding and to control the bleeding. May also be used to obtain specimens for bacteriologic, histologic, and cytologic evaluations
Ventilation–perfusion (VQ) scan	Useful in patients suspected of having hemoptysis due to pulmonary embolism or infarct
Pulmonary arteriography	Selective angiography may locate the site of bleeding, and bronchial artery embolization may be used to control bleeding in cases of massive hemoptysis
Test of sputum for occult blood	If there is doubt that the sputum contains blood
Arterial blood gases	To assess oxygenation, ventilation, and circulation in patients with signs of hemodynamic instability or respiratory impairment
Urinalysis	If vasculitis or Goodpasture's syndrome is suspected

Further reading

Corder R. Hemoptysis. Emergency Medicine Clinics of North America 2003;21: 421–435.

Jean-Baptiste E. Clinical assessment and management of massive hemoptysis. Critical Care Medicine 2000;28: 1642–1647.

Tasker AD, Flower CDR. Imaging the airways: hemoptysis, bronchiectasis, and small airways disease. Clinics in Chest Medicine 1999;20: 761–773.

33 HIRSUTISM

General Discussion

Hirsutism is defined as the presence of excessive coarse terminal hair in a pattern not normal in the female in areas such as the face, chest, or upper abdomen. This disorder is a sign of increased androgen action on hair follicles, which may result from increased levels of endogenous or exogenous androgens or may result from increased sensitivity of hair follicles to normal levels of circulating androgens.

When evaluating hirsutism, it is important to determine whether hirsutism exists alone or whether virilization is also present. This distinction is important as virilization may reflect a serious underlying pathologic condition such as malignancy. Virilization presents with a wide range of signs of androgen excess such as acne, hirsutism, frontotemporal balding, amenorrhea, oligomenorrhea, deepening of the voice, and clitoromegaly.

The most common triggering factor for hirsutism is excess androgen production. Although androgens may come from an exogenous source, androgen excess is most commonly endogenous. The two primary sources of endogenous androgens are the adrenal glands and the ovaries. Adrenal causes include congenital adrenal hyperplasia, Cushing's syndrome, or tumors. Ovarian causes include polycystic ovary syndrome and tumors.

Medications Associated with Hirsutism

Anabolic steroids

Danazol

Methyldopa

Metoclopramide

Phenothiazines

Progestins (especially levonorgestrel, norethindrone, and norgestrel)

Reserpine

Testosterone

Causes of Hirsutism

Congenital adrenal hyperplasia

Cushing's syndrome

Exogenous pharmacologic source of androgens

Familial hirsutism

Idiopathic

Medications

Polycystic ovary syndrome

Tumor (ovarian, adrenal, or pituitary)

Key Historical Features

✓ Onset and extent of hair growth

✓ Past medical history

✓ Menstrual and reproductive history

✓ Medications

✓ Family history

✓ Weight gain

✓ Abdominal symptoms

✓ Breast discharge or galactorrhea

✓ Skin symptoms such as acne, dryness, or striae

✓ Virilization symptoms

Key Physical Findings

✓ Blood pressure, height, weight

✓ Evaluation of hair distribution and characteristics

✓ Skin evaluation (for acanthosis nigricans, acne, striae, hyperpigmentation)

✓ Breast exam for nipple discharge or galactorrhea

✓ Abdominal examination for masses

✓ Pelvic examination for masses

✓ Signs of Cushing's syndrome

✓ Signs of virilization

Suggested Work-Up

Serum testosterone, serum 17a-hydroxyprogesterone (17-OHP), and DHEA sulfate (DHEAS)	To evaluate for ovarian and adrenal tumors and adult-onset adrenal hyperplasia
Serum prolactin	To evaluate for pituitary tumors
TSH	To evaluate for thyroid dysfunction

Fasting serum glucose	To evaluate for insulin resistance in patients suspected of having polycystic ovary syndrome

Additional Work-Up

ACTH stimulation test	When Cushing's syndrome or adult-onset congenital adrenal hyperplasia is suspected
Glucose tolerance test	In patients with suspected polycystic ovary syndrome with elevated fasting serum glucose
CT of the abdomen and pelvis	To assess the adrenal glands and ovaries in patients whose history, physical, or laboratory evaluation suggest the presence of a virilizing tumor

Further reading

Gilchrist VJ, Hecht BR. A practical approach to hirsutism. American Family Physician 1995; 52: 1837–1846.

Hunter MH, Carek PJ. Evaluation and treatment of women with hirsutism. American Family Physician 2003;67: 2565–2572.

Leung AK, Robson WL. Hirsutism. International Journal of Dermatology 1993;32: 773–777.

Plouffe L. Disorders of excessive hair growth in the adolescent. Obstetrics and Gynecology Clinics 2000;27: 79–99.

Redmond GP, Bergfeld WF. Diagnostic approach to androgen disorders in women: acne, hirsutism, and alopecia. Cleveland Clinic Journal of Medicine 1990;57: 423–427.

Speroff L, Glass RH, Kase NG, eds. Clinical gynecologic endocrinology and infertility, 6th ed. Baltimore: Lippincott Williams & Wilkins; 1999: 529–556.

General Discussion

The three pathophysiological mechanisms for hypercalcemia are increased bone resorption, increased gastrointestinal absorption of calcium, and decreased renal excretion of calcium. Increased bone resorption accounts for most cases of hypercalcemia and is seen in both primary hyperparathyroidism and malignancy. Increased gastrointestinal absorption of calcium usually is mediated by vitamin D through an increase in the production of 1,25 dihydroxyvitamin D, a mechanism seen in lymphomas and granulomatous disease. Decreased renal excretion of calcium is rare but may be caused by medications such as diuretics and lithium that affect the renal handling of calcium.

Concentrations of calcium are highly modulated through the actions of parathyroid hormone (PTH), calcitonin, and vitamin D acting on target organs such as bone, kidney, and the gastrointestinal tract. Primary hyperparathyroidism represents the leading cause of hypercalcemia, and malignancy is the second leading cause. Together, they account for more than 90% of the cases of hypercalcemia.

Primary hyperparathyroidism is usually caused by a single adenoma of the parathyroid gland. Glandular hyperplasia, multiple adenomas, and parathyroid malignancy are less common. The hypercalcemia of malignancy is caused by increased bone resorption from skeletal metastases or the production of parathyroid hormone related peptide (PTHrP) that stimulates osteoclasts.

Since low albumin levels can affect the total calcium level, the evaluation of hypercalcemia begins with the calculation of the corrected calcium level using the following formula:

$$\text{Corrected calcium} = ((4.0 \text{ g per dL} - [\text{plasma albumin}]) \times 0.8) + [\text{serum calcium}]$$

If the patient is on any medications known to be associated with hypercalcemia, the causative medications should be stopped and the calcium levels rechecked. If the patient is not on any of these medications or if the calcium level remains high, the work-up for hypercalcemia may begin. The serum PTH level helps guide the evaluation of hypercalcemia. PTH is elevated in primary hyperparathyroidism and suppressed in malignancy-associated hypercalcemia. The remainder of the diagnostic evaluation is outlined below.

Medications and Ingestions Associated with Hypercalcemia

Betel nuts

Calcium

Calcium and vitamin D (milk alkali syndrome)

Dialysate calcium

Ganciclovir

Growth hormone therapy

Lithium

Manganese

Parenteral nutrition

Tamoxifen

Theophylline

Thiazide diuretics

Thyroid hormone excess

Vitamin A

Vitamin D

Causes of Hypercalcemia

Endocrine/metabolic disorders

- Familial hypocalciuric hypercalcemia
- Hyperthyroidism
- Hypoadrenalism
- Hypophosphatasia
- Lactase deficiency
- Multiple endocrine neoplasia types I and IIa
- Pheochromocytoma
- Primary hyperparathyroidism
- Vipoma
- William's syndrome

Granulomatous disease

- Bartonella (cat-scratch disease)
- Berylliosis
- Blastomyces
- Candidiasis
- Coccidioidomycosis
- Cryptococcus
- Cytomegalovirus
- Histoplasmosis
- HIV/AIDS-associated
- Leprosy
- Nocardia

- Pneumocystis
- Pulmonary eosinophilic granuloma
- Sarcoidosis
- Silicone injections
- Talc
- Tuberculosis
- Wegener granulomatosis

Immobilization
- Adolescence
- Guillain–Barré
- Paget's disease
- Thyrotoxicosis
- Whole-body cast

Inflammatory disease
- Acute rheumatic fever
- Crohn's disease
- Richter's syndrome
- Systemic lupus erythematosus
- Wegener granulomatosis

Malignancy
- Leukemia
- Lymphoma
- Multiple myeloma
- Solid tumors (lung cancer, breast cancer, renal cell carcinoma, prostate cancer, cholangiocarcinoma, colon cancer, and squamous cell carcinoma of the head and neck)

Medications

Parathyroid hormone-related

Renal disease
- Renal failure (recovery phase, rhabdomyolysis)
- Tertiary hyperparathyroidism

Key Historical Features

✓ Age

✓ Sex

✓ Risk factors for malignancy

✓ Past medical history

✓ Medications

✓ Family history (especially of hypercalcemia-associated conditions)

✓ Constitutional symptoms

- Fatigue
- Itching
- Muscle weakness
- Polydipsia
- Polyuria

✓ Gastrointestinal symptoms

- Abdominal pain
- Anorexia
- Constipation
- Nausea and vomiting

✓ Neurologic symptoms

- Coma
- Confusion
- Impaired concentration and memory
- Lethargy
- Seizure

Key Physical Findings

✓ Blood pressure for evidence of hypertension

✓ General examination, especially for evidence of malignancy

✓ Head and neck exam focusing on the thyroid and parathyroid glands

✓ Abdominal exam, especially for the possibility of ulcer, pancreatic tumor, or pancreatitis

✓ Neurological exam to test for proximal muscle weakness, easy fatigability, and muscle atrophy

Suggested Work-Up

Serum calcium	To determine the calcium level
Serum albumin	Used to calculate the corrected calcium
PTH	Increased in primary hyperparathyroidism and suppressed in malignancy-associated hypercalcemia

Serum phosphorus	To evaluate for hyperphosphatemia
Serum electrolytes	To assess metabolic status
BUN and creatinine	To evaluate renal function
Electrocardiogram	To evaluate for shortened QTc intervals and the presence of the Osborn, or J wave

Additional Work-Up

If the PTH level is normal or high:

Twenty-four-hour urinary calcium level	Urinary calcium levels are low in patients with familial hypocalciuric hypercalcemia and are high or normal in patients with hyperparathyroidism

If the PTH level is suppressed (malignancy work-up should be guided by symptoms):

PTHrP	Elevated in adenocarcinomas and squamous cell carcinomas
Alkaline phosphatase	Elevated alkaline phosphatase is suggestive of osteolytic hypercalcemia of malignancy
Serum and urine protein electrophoresis	To evaluate for multiple myeloma
Calcitriol	May be elevated in lymphoma or granulomatous diseases

If malignancy work-up is negative:

TSH	To evaluate for hyperthyroidism
Cortisol level	To evaluate for adrenal insufficiency
Insulin-like growth factor I and pituitary MRI	If acromegaly is suspected

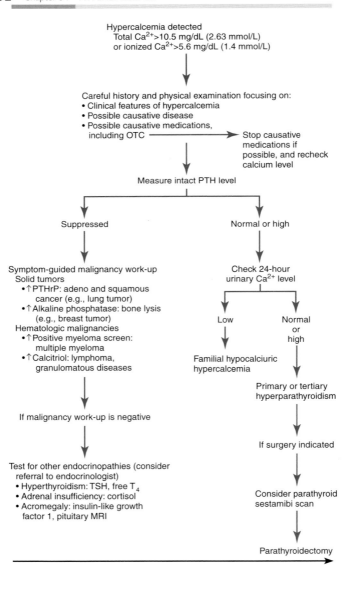

Hypercalcemia detected
Total Ca^{2+} >10.5 mg/dL (2.63 mmol/L)
or ionized Ca^{2+} >5.6 mg/dL (1.4 mmol/L)

Careful history and physical examination focusing on:
- Clinical features of hypercalcemia
- Possible causative disease
- Possible causative medications,
  including OTC → Stop causative
  medications if
  possible, and recheck
  calcium level

Measure intact PTH level

Suppressed

Normal or high

Symptom-guided malignancy work-up
Solid tumors
- ↑PTHrP: adeno and squamous
  cancer (e.g., lung tumor)
- ↑Alkaline phosphatase: bone lysis
  (e.g., breast tumor)
Hematologic malignancies
- ↑Positive myeloma screen:
  multiple myeloma
- ↑Calcitriol: lymphoma,
  granulomatous diseases

Check 24-hour
urinary Ca^{2+} level

Low

Normal
or
high

Familial hypocalciuric
hypercalcemia

Primary or tertiary
hyperparathyroidism

If malignancy work-up is negative

If surgery indicated

Test for other endocrinopathies (consider
referral to endocrinologist)
- Hyperthyroidism: TSH, free T_4
- Adrenal insufficiency: cortisol
- Acromegaly: insulin-like growth
  factor 1, pituitary MRI

Consider parathyroid
sestamibi scan

Parathyroidectomy

Further reading

Ariyan CE, Sosa JA. Assessment and management of patients with abnormal calcium. Critical Care Medicine 2004;32(4Suppl): S146–S154.

Barri YM, Knochel JP. Hypercalcemia and electrolyte disturbances in malignancy. Hematology/Oncology Clinics of North America 1996;10: 775–790.

Carroll MF, Schade DS. A practical approach to hypercalcemia. American Family Physician 2003;67: 1959–1966.

Deftos LJ. Hypercalcemia in malignant and inflammatory diseases. Endocrinology and Metabolism Clinics 2002;31: 141–158.

Taniegra ED. Hyperparathyroidism. American Family Physician 2004;69: 333–339.

Figure 34-1. Diagnostic algorithm for the evaluation of hypercalcemia. Primary hyperparathyroidism and malignancy account for more than 90% of cases. Intact PTH will be suppressed in cases of malignancy-associated hypercalcemia, except for the extremely rare parathyroid carcinoma. The physician can conclude diagnostic testing and treat the causative disorder once a final diagnosis step has been reached. (Ca^{2+} = calcium; MRI = magnetic resonance imaging; OTC = over-the-counter; PTH = parathyroid hormone; PTHrP = parathyroid hormone-related peptide; T4 = free thyroxine; TSH = thyroid-stimulating hormone.)

35 HYPERCOAGULABLE STATES

General Discussion

Hypercoagulable conditions are classified as primary (an inherited condition) or secondary (an acquired state). The inherited disorders include factor V Leiden, prothrombin G20210A gene mutation, hyperhomocysteinemia, elevated factor VIII level, and the deficiencies of antithrombin, protein C, and protein S. Acquired hypercoagulable conditions include the antiphospholipid syndrome (lupus anticoagulant and anticardiolipin antibody), hyperhomocysteinemia, and the commonly known thrombosis risk factors of pregnancy, cancer, and estrogen-containing medications.

There is no standardized approach to screening patients for hypercoagulability. The cost-effectiveness of performing the laboratory examination is unknown, and the work-up typically is expensive. Most clinicians take into consideration patient risk factors when deciding upon the need for an extensive work-up. Any one of the following indicators typically calls for further evaluation: thrombosis at a young age (less than 50 years), family history of thrombosis, recurrent thrombosis, idiopathic thrombosis, and thrombosis at an unusual site such as mesenteric, cerebral, or portal veins.

Risk Factors for Venous Thrombosis

Previous venous thromboembolism

Inherited or acquired thrombophilias

Surgical and nonsurgical trauma

Immobilization

Malignancy

Pregnancy

Oral contraceptive and other estrogen use

Advancing age

Heart disease

Leg paralysis

Suggested Work-Up

CBC	To screen for myeloproliferative disease
Activated PTT	To screen for lupus anticoagulant
Anticardiolipin antibody	
Anti-thrombin III	

Factor V Leiden (gene mutation)

Factor VIII level

Homocysteine level

Lupus anticoagulant

Protein C

Protein S

Prothrombin G20210A

Further reading

Alpert MA. Homocysteine, atherosclerosis, and thrombosis. Southern Medical Journal 1999; 92: 858–865.

Barger AP, Hurley R. Evaluation of the hypercoagulable state: whom to screen, how to test and treat. Postgraduate Medicine 2000;108: 59–66.

DeStefano V, Finazzi G, Mannucci PM. Inherited thrombophilia: pathogenesis, clinical syndromes, and management. Blood 1996;87: 531.

Faioni EM, Valsecchi C, Palla A, et al. Free protein S deficiency is risk factor for venous thrombosis. Thrombosis and Haemostasis 1997;78: 1343.

Federman DG, Kirsner RS. An update on hypercoagulable disorders. Archives of Internal Medicine 2001;161: 1051–1056.

Koster T, Blann AD, Briet E, et al. Role of clotting factor VIII in effect of von Willebrand factor on occurrence of deep-vein thrombosis. Lancet 1995;345: 152–155.

Poort SR, Rosendaal FR, Reitsma PH, et al. A common genetic variant in the 3'-untranslated region of the prothrombin gene is associated with elevated plasma prothrombin levels and an increase in thrombosis. Thrombosis and Haemostasis 1997;78: 1430–1433.

Tait RC, Walker ID, Retsma PH, et al. Prevalence of protein C deficiency in the healthy population. Thrombosis and Haemostasis 1995;73: 87.

General Discussion

Hyperkalemia is defined as a serum potassium concentration greater than 5.0 mEq/L and can become life threatening when the potassium concentration rises above 6.5 mEq/L. Hyperkalemia often is asymptomatic, but may affect normal cardiac conduction, producing characteristic EKG changes which are outlined below. Although there is no clear correlation between the degree of hyperkalemia and the likelihood of life-threatening arrhythmias, an arrhythmia is more likely to occur if the serum potassium concentration increases rapidly. All patients with a serum potassium concentration greater than 6.0 mEq/L should be considered at risk for cardiac arrhythmias.

All disorders of potassium occur because of abnormal handling of potassium in one of three ways: problems with potassium intake, problems with potassium excretion, or problems with distribution of potassium between the intracellular and extracellular spaces.

The primary source of potassium intake is through food. Generally speaking, fruits and vegetables have the highest concentrations of potassium. Salt substitutes represent a commonly overlooked source of dietary potassium. Under normal circumstances, 80–90% of dietary potassium is eliminated via renal excretion.

The organ systems affected by hyperkalemia are cardiac, neuromuscular, and gastrointestinal. Symptoms may include not feeling well, fatigue, paresthesias, muscle weakness, or muscle cramps.

Over 80% of clinical episodes of hyperkalemia are caused by impaired potassium excretion caused by renal insufficiency. Patients with acute renal failure are at greater risk for life-threatening complications from hyperkalemia because the potassium level rises more rapidly.

Medications and Supplements Associated with Hyperkalemia

Alpha blockers

Amino acids

- Arginine
- Epsilon-aminocaproic acid
- Lysine

Angiotensin converting enzyme (ACE) inhibitors

Angiotensin receptor blockers

Azole antifungals

Beta blockers

Cyclosporine

Digoxin

Eplerenone

Ethinyl estradiol/drospirenone

Herbal remedies and nutritional supplements

- Alfalfa
- Dandelion
- Hawthorn berries
- Horsetail
- Lily of the valley
- Milkweed
- Nettle
- Noni juice
- Siberian ginseng

Heparin

NSAIDs

Penicillin G potassium

Pentamidine

Potassium-sparing diuretics

- Amiloride
- Spironolactone
- Triamterene

Potassium supplements

Succinylcholine

Tacrolimus

Trimethoprim-sulfamethoxazole

Causes of Hyperkalemia

Acidosis

Addison's disease

AIDS

Amyloidosis

Burns

Congenital adrenal hyperplasia

Familial hyperkalemic periodic paralysis

Fluoride toxicity

Hereditary enzyme deficiencies

Hypertonicity due to uncontrolled diabetes

Infusion of packed red blood cells

Insulin deficiency or resistance

Pseudohyperkalemia

- Fist clenching with tourniquet in place
- Hemolysis
- Leukocytosis (white blood cell count >100,000/mm^3)
- Thrombocytosis (platelets >1,000,000/mm^3)

Pseudohypoaldosteronism

Renal failure (acute and chronic)

Renal insufficiency

Renal transplantation

Rhabdomyolysis

Selective hypoaldosteronism

Sickle cell anemia

Systemic lupus erythematosus

Trauma

Tumor lysis syndrome

Type 4 renal tubular acidosis

Key Historical Features

✓ Generally not feeling well

✓ Fatigue

✓ Muscle weakness

✓ Paresthesias

✓ Muscle cramps

✓ Gastrointestinal symptoms such as constipation

✓ History of salt substitute intake

✓ Past medical history, especially renal insufficiency

✓ Medications

✓ Herbal and dietary supplement use

✓ Family history

Key Physical Findings

✓ Vital signs

✓ Cardiac examination for arrhythmias

✓ Gastrointestinal examination

✓   Neurologic examination for muscle weakness or decreased deep tendon reflexes

Suggested Work-Up

EKG	To evaluate the effect of hyperkalemia on the myocardium. May reveal peaked T waves, widened QRS complexes, increased PR interval, AV conduction blockade with a slow idioventricular rhythm, or ventricular fibrillation
Serum chemistry	To measure electrolytes and evaluate for acidosis
BUN and creatinine	To evaluate renal function
Spot urine for potassium, creatinine, and osmoles (U_{Cr}/S_{Cr})	To calculate the fractional excretion of potassium (FEK): $(U_{K}/S_{K}) \times 100\%$
	FEK <10% indicates renal etiology
	FEK >10% indicates extrarenal etiology
Morning serum cortisol level	To evaluate for Addison's disease

Additional Work-Up

Adrenocorticotropic hormone stimulation test	If the morning serum cortisol level is low to evaluate for Addison's disease
Measurement of plasma and serum potassium concentrations	If pseudohyperkalemia is suspected

Further reading

Gennari FJ. Disorders of potassium homeostasis; hypokalemia and hyperkalemia. Critical Care Clinics 2002;18: 273–288.

Hollander-Rodriguez JC, Calvert JF. Hyperkalemia. American Family Physician 2006;73: 283–290.

Mandal AK. Hypokalemia and hyperkalemia. Medical Clinics of North America 1997;81: 611–639.

Schaefer TJ, Wolford RW. Disorders of potassium. Emergency Medicine Clinics of North America 2005;23: 723–747.

Weiner ID, Wingo CS. Hyperkalemia: a potential silent killer. Journal of the American Society of Nephrology 1998;9: 1535–1543.

General Discussion

Hypernatremia is defined as a serum sodium concentration exceeding 145 mEq/L. In contrast to hyponatremia, which usually results from a defect in renal water handling, the primary defect in hypernatremia is impaired water intake. Hypernatremia represents a deficit of water in relation to the body's sodium stores, which may result from a net water loss or a hypertonic sodium gain. Unlike hyponatremia, hypernatremia always represents a hyperosmolar state. The majority of cases of hypernatremia result from a net water loss.

Hypernatremia is rarely found in an alert patient who has access to water and a normal thirst mechanism. Sustained hypernatremia occurs when thirst is impaired or access to water is limited, so the groups at highest risk are patients with altered mental status, intubated patients, elderly persons, and infants. In elderly persons, hypernatremia is usually associated with infirmity or febrile illness. Hypernatremia is also more common after age 60 because increased age is associated with decreased osmotic stimulation of thirst and decreased maximal urinary concentration.

Signs and symptoms of hypernatremia reflect central nervous system dysfunction and are most prominent when the increase in the serum sodium concentration is large and occurs rapidly. Elderly patients generally have few symptoms until the serum sodium concentration exceeds 160 mmol per liter. Brain shrinkage induced by hypernatremia can cause vascular rupture, with cerebral bleeding and permanent neurologic damage or death.

Central diabetes insipidus results from deficient vasopressin secretion while nephrogenic diabetes insipidus results from end organ hyporesponsiveness to vasopressin. Diabetes insipidus is associated with variable degrees of polyuria and an inability to concentrate urine maximally.

Medications Associated with Hypernatremia

Amphotericin B

Demeclocycline

Foscarnet

Lactulose

Lithium

Loop diuretics

Methoxyflurane

Vasopressin receptor antagonists

Causes of Hypernatremia

Net water loss

- Burns
- Excessive sweating
- Gastrointestinal losses (vomiting, diarrhea, nasogastric suctioning, enterocutaneous fistula, lactulose)
- Hypothalamic disorder (primary hypodipsia, resetting of osmostat)
- Insensible losses
- Intrinsic renal disease
- Loop diuretics
- Nephrogenic diabetes insipidus (hypercalcemia, hypokalemia, medications, medullary cystic disease)
- Neurogenic diabetes insipidus (trauma, encephalopathy, tumor, cyst, tuberculosis, sarcoidosis, histiocytosis, idiopathic, aneurysm, meningitis, encephalitis, Guillain–Barré syndrome, ethanol ingestion)
- Osmotic diuresis with glucose, urea, or mannitol
- Third space fluid losses (bowel obstruction, ileus, pancreatitis)

Hypertonic sodium gain

- Cushing's syndrome
- Hypertonic dialysis
- Hypertonic feeding
- Hypertonic sodium chloride infusion
- Intrauterine injection of hypertonic saline
- Primary hyperaldosteronism
- Sea water ingestion
- Sodium bicarbonate infusion
- Sodium chloride ingestion

Key Historical Features

✓ Symptoms of hypernatremia (muscle weakness, lethargy, irritability, restlessness, confusion, coma)

✓ Fever

✓ Nausea or vomiting

✓ Presence of thirst

✓ Polyuria and polydipsia

✓ Recent fluid losses

✓ Recent intravenous or intrauterine fluid administration

✓ Past medical history, especially any neurologic disease

✓ Medications

✓ Functional status and ability to obtain drinking water

Key Physical Findings

✓ Vital signs

✓ Assessment of volume status

✓ Head and neck examination to evaluate for dry mucous membranes

✓ Cardiac examination for tachycardia

✓ Neurologic examination for hyperreflexia, spasticity, or weakness

Suggested Work-Up

Urine osmolality and urine sodium concentration	Low urine sodium and a maximally concentrated urine (>700 mmol/kg) suggests extrarenal hypotonic fluid losses. When losses are renal in origin, the urine osmolality is inappropriately low.
	With diuretics, osmotic diuresis, or salt wasting, the urine osmolality is isotonic at approximately 300 mmol/kg. Patients with urine osmolality of less than 200 mmol/kg usually have some form of diabetes insipidus.
	A urine osmolality of less than 150 mmol/kg in the setting of hypertonicity and polyuria is diagnostic of diabetes insipidus.

Additional Work-Up

Vasopressin administration	If diabetes insipidus is suspected to differentiate the hypothalamic and nephrogenic forms
Serum potassium and serum calcium	If nephrogenic diabetes insipidus is suggested by the diagnostic evaluation outlined above

Further reading

Adrogue HJ, Madias NE. Hypernatremia. New England Journal of Medicine 2000;
    342: 1493–1499.

Fall PJ. Hyponatremia and hypernatremia: a systematic approach to causes and their
    correction. Postgraduate Medicine 2000;107: 75–82.

Fried LF, Palevsky PM. Hyponatremia and hypernatremia. Medical Clinics of North America
    1997;81: 585–609.

Kumar S, Berl T. Sodium. Lancet 1998;352: 220–228.

38 HYPERTENSION

General Discussion

The relationship between blood pressure and the risk of cardiovascular disease is continuous, consistent, and independent of other risk factors. As the blood pressure rises, so does the risk of myocardial infarction, heart failure, stroke, and kidney disease. For individuals 40–70 years of age, each increment of 20 mmHg in systolic blood pressure or 10 mmHg in diastolic blood pressure doubles the risk of cardiovascular disease across the entire blood pressure range from 115/75 to 185/115 mmHg.

The JNC 7 report has introduced a new classification that includes the term "prehypertension" for those with blood pressures ranging from 120 to 139 mmHg systolic and/or 80 to 89 mmHg diastolic. Normal blood pressure is defined as less than 120/80 mmHg.

The evaluation of patients with hypertension has three objectives. First, the patient's lifestyle and cardiovascular risk factors should be assessed. Second, identifiable causes of hypertension should be identified. Third, the presence or absence of target organ damage and cardiovascular disease should be assessed.

Medications Associated with Hypertension

Adrenal steroids

Anorectics

Cyclosporin

Decongestants

Erythropoietin

NSAIDs

Oral contraceptives

Over-the-counter medicines (bitter orange, ephedra, ma huang)

Tacrolimus

Identifiable Causes of Hypertension

Chronic kidney disease

Chronic steroid therapy

Coarctation of the aorta

Cushing's disease

Obstructive sleep apnea

Parathyroid disease

Pheochromocytoma

Primary aldosteronism
Renovascular disease
Thyroid disease

Suggested Work-Up

EKG	To evaluate for left ventricular hypertrophy or prior myocardial infarction
Urinalysis	To evaluate for renal disease/proteinuria
Hemoglobin and hematocrit	To evaluate for anemia or polycythemia
Serum potassium	To evaluate for primary aldosteronism
Serum creatinine	To evaluate for renal function
Serum calcium	To evaluate for parathyroid disease
Fasting blood glucose	To evaluate for glucose intolerance or diabetes mellitus
Fasting lipid panel, including LDL, HDL, and triglycerides	To evaluate for dyslipidemia

Additional Work-Up

According to JNC 7, more extensive testing for identifiable causes is not generally indicated unless blood pressure control is not achieved or the clinical and routine laboratory evaluation strongly suggests a secondary cause of hypertension. Signs and symptoms that may suggest a secondary cause include vascular bruits, symptoms of catecholamine excess, or unprovoked hypokalemia.

Renal ultrasound	In patients with elevated creatinine or abnormal urinalysis on initial screen
CT angiogram	In patients suspected of having coarctation of the aorta (decreased pressure in the lower extremities or delayed or absent femoral arterial pulses)

Dexamethasone suppression test	In patients suspected of having Cushing's disease (truncal obesity, glucose intolerance, striae)
Drug screening	In patients suspected of having drug-induced hypertension
24-hour urinary metanephrine and normetanephrine	In patients suspected of having pheochromocytoma (labile hypertension or paroxysms of hypertension accompanied by headache, palpitations, pallor, and perspiration)
24-hour urinary aldosterone	In patients suspected of having primary aldosteronism (unprovoked hypokalemia on initial screen)
Doppler flow study or MRI angiography or ACE-inhibitor-enhanced renal scan	In patients suspected of having renovascular hypertension (early onset of hypertension, abdominal bruit, accelerated hypertension, recurrent flash pulmonary edema, renal failure of uncertain etiology, or acute renal failure precipitated by therapy with an ACE inhibitor or angiotensin receptor blocker)
Sleep study	In patients suspected of having sleep apnea
TSH	In patients suspected of having thyroid disease
Serum PTH	In patients suspected of having parathyroid disease (hypercalcemia on initial screen)

Further reading

Lewington S, Clarke R, Qizilbash N, et al. Age-specific relevance of usual blood pressure to vascular mortality: A meta-analysis of individual data for one million adults in 61 prospective studies. Lancet 2002;360: 1903–1913.

Philips LS, Branch WT, Cook CB, et al. Clinical inertia. Annals of Internal Medicine 2001; 135: 825–834.

The seventh report of the joint national committee on prevention, detection, evaluation, and treatment of high blood pressure. Journal of the American Medical Association 2003; 289: 2560–2572.

General Discussion

Hyperthyroidism is a hypermetabolic state that results from excess synthesis and release of thyroid hormone, usually from the thyroid gland. The overall incidence of subclinical and overt hyperthyroidism is estimated to be 0.05–0.1% in the general population. Hyperthyroidism occurs in all age groups and is more common in women than in men. Graves' disease is the most common cause of hyperthyroidism, causing 60–80% of cases. However, toxic nodular goiter is the most common cause of hyperthyroidism in the elderly.

Hyperthyroidism may present as a spectrum from asymptomatic, subclinical hyperthyroidism to life-threatening thyroid storm. Subclinical hyperthyroidism is diagnosed in asymptomatic patients with low thyroid stimulating hormone (TSH) but normal free T4 and free T3. Clinical hyperthyroidism presents with the typical signs and symptoms outlined below.

Elderly patients often present a diagnostic challenge as they may present with lone symptoms or atypical presentations. They may present with negative symptoms such as depressive symptoms, lethargy, or apathetic facies. Elderly patients also may present with only a small goiter, weight loss, worsening of underlying cardiovascular disease, or new-onset atrial fibrillation.

Medications Associated with Hyperthyroidism

Amiodarone

Campath 1-H monoclonal antibody

Highly active antiretroviral therapy (HAART)

Interferon-α

Lithium

Causes of Hyperthyroidism

Factitious hyperthyroidism

Graves' disease

Iodine-induced hyperthyroidism (iodine ingestion, radiographic contrast, amiodarone)

Lymphocytic thyroiditis (Hashimoto's thyroiditis)

Medication-induced thyroiditis

Metastatic thyroid cancer

Ovarian tumors (struma ovarii)

Pituitary adenoma secreting TSH

Postpartum thyroiditis

Toxic adenoma

Toxic multinodular goiter

Trophoblastic tumor

Key Historical Features

✓ Constitutional symptoms
- Anxiety
- Excessive perspiration
- Fatigue
- Heat intolerance
- Nervousness
- Pruritis
- Thirst
- Weight loss

✓ Cardiac symptoms
- Anginal symptoms
- Exertional dyspnea
- Orthopnea
- Palpitations
- Reduced exercise tolerance

✓ Pulmonary symptoms
- Dyspnea

✓ Gastrointestinal symptoms
- Difficulty swallowing
- Dyspepsia
- Frequent bowel movements
- Nausea and vomiting
- Rapid intestinal transit time

✓ Genitourinary
- Erectile dysfunction
- Nocturia
- Urinary frequency

✓ Ophthalmologic
- Diplopia

- Eye irritation or dryness
- Excessive tearing
- Pain with eye movements
- Visual blurring

✓ Reproductive symptoms

- Amenorrhea
- Decreased libido
- Gynecomastia
- Infertility
- Menometrorrhagia
- Oligomenorrhea
- Spider angiomas

✓ Neuromuscular symptoms

- Fatigability
- Generalized weakness
- Proximal muscle weakness

✓ Psychiatric symptoms

- Altered mental status
- Emotional lability
- Insomnia
- Memory loss
- Nightmares and vivid dreams
- Poor attention span
- Restlessness

✓ Past medical history

✓ Recent pregnancy

✓ Smoking

✓ Family history

Key Physical Findings

✓ Vital signs, especially tachycardia or hypertension

✓ Skin and hair

- Warm, smooth, velvety skin
- Skin hyperpigmentation
- Palmar erythema
- Pretibial myxedema

- • Fine, brittle scalp hair
- • Diffuse alopecia
- • Nail changes (onycholysis)

✓ Eyes

- • Exophthalmos
- • Proptosis
- • Lid lag
- • Infrequent blinking
- • Vasodilation of the conjunctiva
- • Lid or periorbital edema
- • Papilledema

✓ Thyroid

- • Diffuse enlargement
- • Single nodule
- • Multinodular goiter
- • Bruit

✓ Cardiovascular

- • Tachycardia
- • Bounding pulses
- • Rapid and brisk carotid upstroke
- • Systolic flow murmurs
- • Atrial arrhythmias such as atrial fibrillation or atrial flutter

✓ Pulmonary

- • Tachypnea

✓ Musculoskeletal

- • Decreased muscle strength
- • Decreased muscle volume
- • Muscle atrophy
- • Muscle weakness, especially proximal

✓ Neurological

- • Brisk reflexes
- • Fidgeting
- • Nervousness
- • Hyperactivity and rapid speech

Suggested Work-Up

TSH	To evaluate thyroid function
Radionuclide uptake scan	To distinguish Graves' disease from thyroiditis and provide anatomic information

Additional Work-Up

Thyroglobulin level	May help distinguish Graves' disease (elevated thyroglobulin) from factitious thyrotoxicosis (decreased thyroglobulin)
Thyroid peroxidase antibodies	Elevated in Graves' disease and lymphocytic thyroiditis

Further reading

Ginsberg J. Diagnosis and management of Graves' disease. Canadian Medical Association Journal 2003;168: 575–585.

McKeown NJ, Tews MC, Gossain VV, et al. Hyperthyroidism. Emergency Medicine Clinics of North America 2005;23: 669–685.

Reid JR, Wheeler SF. Hyperthyroidism: diagnosis and treatment. American Family Physician 2005;72: 623–630.

40 HYPOGLYCEMIA

General Discussion

Symptoms of hypoglycemia begin at plasma glucose levels of approximately 60 mg/dL, and impairment of nervous system function begins at approximately 50 mg/dL. Clinical hypoglycemia is identified by modified Whipple's criteria: (1) CNS symptoms, including confusion, aberrant behavior, or coma; (2) a simultaneous blood glucose level equal to or less than 40 mg/dL; and (3) relief of these symptoms by the administration of glucose.

The causes of hypoglycemia may be categorized into three main groups for the purposes of evaluation. These categories are medication- or toxin-induced hypoglycemia, disorders associated with fasting hypoglycemia, and disorders associated with postprandial hypoglycemia. Each of these categories is outlined in detail below. The list of medications associated with hypoglycemia is also listed below.

Four simultaneous criteria should be present to establish the diagnosis of insulinoma:

1. Blood glucose less than 40 mg/dL
2. Symptoms of neuroglycopenia
3. Plasma insulin greater than 5 muU/mL
4. Plasma C-peptide greater than 0.6 ng/mL

Medications Associated with Hypoglycemia

ACE inhibitors

Acetazolamide

Acetohexamide

Aspirin

Azapropazone

Benzodiazepines

Buformin

Carbutamide

Chloroquine

Chlorpromazine

Chlorpropamide

Cibenzoline

Cimetidine

Ciprofloxacin

Clipizide

Cycloheptolamide

Dicumarol

Diphenhydramine

Disopyramide

Doxepin

Ecstasy (MDMA)

Enflurane

Ethionamide

Etomidate

Fenoterol

Fluoxetine

Formestane

Furosemide

Glibenclamide

Gliclazide

Glipizide

Glyburide

Haloperidol

Halothane

Herbal extracts

Imipramine

Indomethacin

Insulin

Interferon-α

Isoniazid

Isoxsuprine

Lidocaine

Lithium

Maprotiline

Mefloquine

Metahexamide

Metoprolol

Monoamine oxidase inhibitors

Nadolol

Nefazodone

Octreotide

Orphenadrine

Oxytetracycline

p-aminobenzoic acid (PABA)

p-aminosalicylic acid (PASA)

Paracetamol

Pentamidine

Perhexiline

Phenformin

Phenindione

Phenylbutazone

Phenytoin

Pindolol

Propoxyphene

Propranolol

Quinine

Ranitidine

Ritodrine

Salicylates

Selegiline

Sulfixasol

Sulfonylureas

Sulphadiazine

Sulphadimidine

Sulfamethoxazole

Sulfaphenazole

Terbutaline

Tolazamide

Tolbutamide

Trimethoprim/sulfamethoxazole

Warfarin

Causes of Hypoglycemia

Medications and toxins

- Factitious hyperinsulinism
- Insulin-induced hypoglycemia (excessive insulin dose, severe exercise, or inadequate food intake)
- Sulfonylureas
- Alcohol
- Other medications as listed above
- Vacor (a rodenticide)

- • Toadstool
- • Hypoglycin (present in Caribbean akee fruit)

Disorders associated with fasting hypoglycemia

- • Adrenal insufficiency
- • Chronic kidney disease
- • Insulin autoantibodies
- • Insulin receptor antibodies
- • Insulinoma
- • Liver disease
- • Non-islet cell tumors
- • Pituitary insufficiency

Disorders associated with postprandial hypoglycemia

- • Early type II diabetes
- • Galactosemia
- • Hereditary fructose intolerance
- • Idiopathic postprandial hypoglycemia
- • Postgastrectomy hypoglycemia

Key Historical Features

✓ Headaches

✓ Fatigue

✓ Diaphoresis

✓ Weakness

✓ Confusion

✓ Difficulty speaking

✓ Blurred vision

✓ Palpitations

✓ Neuromuscular symptoms

✓ Nervousness

✓ Slurred speech

✓ Difficulty concentrating

✓ Aberrant behavior

✓ Focal neurologic signs and symptoms

✓ Seizures

✓ Coma

✓ Past medical history

✓ Medications

Key Physical Findings

✓ Vital signs

✓ Abdominal examination

✓ Neurologic examination

Suggested Work-Up

Measurement of plasma glucose during a symptomatic episode	To establish hypoglycemia as the cause of the patient's symptoms
Meal tolerance test	To determine whether the patient has postprandial hypoglycemia
Basal serum proinsulin	To help rule out insulinoma (usually elevated in patients with insulinoma)
Prolonged fast with frequent determination of glucose, insulin, and C-peptide	To help rule out insulinoma

Additional Work-Up

CT or MR imaging	To localize an insulinoma once the diagnosis has been established
Selective arteriogram, selective arteriogram with calcium stimulation and measurement of insulin in hepatic veins, selective venous sampling of the portal vein, endoscopic ultrasound, and intraoperative ultrasound	To localize an insulinoma once the diagnosis has been established

Further reading

Marks V, Teale JD. Drug-induced hypoglycemia. Endocrinology and Metabolism Clinics 1999;28: 555–577.

Marks V, Teale JD. Hypoglycemia: factitious and felonious. Endocrinology and Metabolism Clinics 1999;28: 579–601.

Pourmotabbed G, Kitabchi AE. Hypoglycemia. Obstetrics and Gynecology Clinics 2001;28: 383–400.

Service FJ. Hypoglycemia. Endocrinology and Metabolism Clinics 1997;26: 937–955.

41 HYPOKALEMIA

General Discussion

Hypokalemia is defined as a serum potassium level less than 3.6 mEq per liter. Hypokalemia has been associated with an increased risk of hypertension, ischemic stroke, hemorrhagic stroke, dysrhythmias, and hospital admissions and deaths due to heart failure and cardiovascular events.

Hypokalemia primarily affects the cardiac, skeletal muscle, gastrointestinal, and renal organ systems. However, patients with hypokalemia are usually asymptomatic. Vague symptoms of fatigue and muscle weakness may be reported.

The etiology of hypokalemia falls into three broad categories: insufficient potassium intake, transcellular shift of potassium from the extracellular to intracellular compartments, or excessive potassium loss. Diuretics are the most common drug-related cause of hypokalemia. Potassium loss via the gastrointestinal tract, usually as a result of diarrhea, is the second most common cause of hypokalemia in developed countries. Inadequate potassium intake is rarely a cause of hypokalemia.

Medications Associated with Hypokalemia

Albuterol

Amphotericin B

Carbenicillin

Cisplatin

Fludrocortisone

Foscarnet

Gentamicin

Hydrocortisone

Loop diuretics

- Bumetanide
- Furosemide
- Torsemide

Penicillin

Theophylline

Thiazide diuretics

- Hydrochlorothiazide
- Metolazone

Verapamil overdose

Causes of Hypokalemia

ACTH-producing bronchogenic tumor

Alcoholism

Barium poisoning

Bartter's syndrome

Caffeine intake

Chewing tobacco containing glycyrrhizic acid

Chloride depletion (metabolic alkalosis)

Chloroquine poisoning

Congenital adrenal hyperplasia

Delirium tremens

Diarrhea

Gastric suctioning

Gitelman's syndrome

Hyperthyroidism

Hypokalemic familial periodic paralysis

Inadequate potassium intake

Insulin poisoning

Laxative abuse

Leukemia

Licorice ingestion containing glycyrrhizic acid

Liddle's syndrome

Magnesium depletion

Medications

Osmotic diuresis (uncontrolled diabetes)

Primary hyperaldosteronism

Renal tubular acidosis types I and II

Secondary hyperaldosteronism

Trauma

Vomiting

11ß-hydroxysteroid dehydrogenase deficiency

Key Historical Features

✓ Muscle weakness

✓ Paralysis

✓ Worsening of weakness with exercise

✓ Vomiting

✓ Diarrhea

✓ Laxative abuse

✓ Licorice intake

✓ Past medical history

✓ Medications

✓ Alcohol abuse

✓ Chewing tobacco

Key Physical Findings

✓ Vital signs

✓ Cardiovascular examination for arrhythmias

✓ Neurologic examination for muscle weakness, especially proximal

Suggested Work-Up

EKG	May reveal U-waves, prolonged PR interval, T-wave inversion, ST segment depression, and QT interval prolongation
Serum chemistry	To evaluate for acidosis and hyperchloremia
BUN and creatinine	To evaluate renal function
Serum magnesium	To evaluate for magnesium depletion

Additional Work-Up

Basal plasma renin activity and plasma aldosterone level	If hypertension is present to evaluate for primary or secondary hyperaldosteronism
Morning urinary pH and ammonium chloride test	To evaluate for type I renal tubular acidosis if hypokalemia and hyperchloremic metabolic acidosis are present
24-hour urinary calcium	To evaluate for hypercalciuria
Flat film of the abdomen or renal ultrasound	To evaluate for nephrocalcinosis or nephrolithiasis

Plasma renin activity, plasma aldosterone level, urinary chloride, and urinary PGE$_2$ levels

If Bartter's syndrome is suspected (short stature, failure to thrive, muscle weakness/cramps, polyuria, and nocturia)

Further reading

Gennari FJ. Disorders of potassium homeostasis: hypokalemia and hyperkalemia. Critical Care Clinics 2002;18: 273–288.

Mandal AK. Hypokalemia and hyperkalemia. Renal disease. Medical Clinics of North America 1997;81: 611–639.

Schaefer TJ, Wolford RW. Disorders of potassium. Emergency Medicine Clinics of North America 2005;23: 723–747.

Webster A, Brady W, Morris F. Recognising signs of danger: ECG changes resulting from an abnormal serum potassium concentration. Emergency Medicine Journal 2002;19: 74–77.

42 HYPONATREMIA

General Discussion

Hyponatremia generally is defined as a plasma sodium level of less than 135 mEq/L. Hyponatremia may lead to significant morbidity and mortality. Most patients with hyponatremia are asymptomatic, and symptoms usually do not appear until the plasma sodium level drops below 120 mEq/L. Symptoms of hyponatremia usually are nonspecific and include headache, nausea, and lethargy. However, neurologic and gastrointestinal symptoms may be present in cases of severe hyponatremia, with the risk of seizure and coma increasing as the sodium level decreases. If the sodium level decreases quickly, symptoms may be present at sodium levels above 120 mEq/L.

The evaluation of hyponatremia begins with a targeted history to evaluate for causes of hyponatremia such as congestive heart failure, renal impairment, liver disease, malignancy, hypothyroidism, or Addison's disease. Hyponatremia is then classified according to the volume status of the patient as hypovolemic, hypervolemic, or euvolemic.

Hypervolemic hyponatremia results in increased total body water and the presence of edema. The three main causes of hypervolemic hyponatremia are congestive heart failure, liver cirrhosis, and renal impairment such as renal failure and nephrotic syndrome.

Differentiating between hypovolemia and euvolemia may be difficult clinically. An elevated hematocrit or a blood urea nitrogen:creatinine ratio greater than 20 may suggest hypovolemia but are not always present. If the patient's volume status is not clear, the measurements of plasma osmolality and urinary sodium concentration are useful for evaluating euvolemic or hypovolemic patients.

Normal plasma osmolality (280–300 mOsm/kg of water) can be seen with pseudohyponatremia or after the absorption of large volumes of hypotonic irrigation fluid during transurethral resection of the prostate. Pseudohyponatremia may occur in the presence of severe hypertriglyceridemia and hyperproteinemia.

Increased plasma osmolality (greater than 300 mOsm/kg of water) in a patient with hyponatremia is caused by severe hyperglycemia.

Decreased plasma osmolality (less than 280 mOsm/kg of water) may occur in a patient who is hypovolemic or euvolemic. The urinary sodium excretion is used to further refine the differential diagnosis.

A high urinary sodium concentration (greater than 30 mmol/L) may result from renal disorders, syndrome of inappropriate antidiuretic hormone secretion (SIADH), reset osmostat syndrome, endocrine deficiencies, medications, or drugs.

A low urinary sodium concentration (less than 30 mmol per L) may result from vomiting, diarrhea, severe burns, acute water overload, or psychogenic polydipsia.

SIADH occurs when antidiuretic hormone is secreted independently of the body's need to conserve water. SIADH is a diagnosis of exclusion but should be suspected when hyponatremia is accompanied by a low serum osmolality with an inappropriately high urine osmolality. The diagnostic criteria for SIADH are:

- Hypotonic hyponatremia
- Urine osmolality greater than 100 mmol/kg
- Absence of extracellular volume depletion
- Normal thyroid and adrenal function
- Normal cardiac, hepatic, and renal function.

Medications Associated with Hyponatremia

Amiodarone

Carbamazepine

Chlorpromazine

Chlorpropamide

Clofibrate

Cyclophosphamide

Haloperidol

Indapamide

Loop diuretics

NSAIDs

Opiates

Oxytocin

Phenothiazines

Selective serotonin reuptake inhibitors

Theophylline

Thiazide diuretics

Tricyclic antidepressants

Vasopressin analogs

Vincristine

Causes of Hyponatremia

Acute intermittent porphyria

Acute psychosis

Addison's disease

Congestive heart failure

Gastrointestinal disorders

- Diarrhea
- Vomiting

Ecstasy ingestion

HIV/AIDS

Hyperproteinemia

Hypertriglyceridemia (severe)

Hypothyroidism

Liver disease

Medications

Neoplasms

- Bronchogenic carcinoma
- Duodenal carcinoma
- Lymphoma
- Mesothelioma
- Pancreatic carcinoma
- Prostate carcinoma
- Thymoma

Neurologic disorders

- Alcohol withdrawal (delirium tremens)
- Brain abscess
- Cerebrovascular accident
- Encephalitis
- Guillain–Barré syndrome
- Hydrocephalus
- Meningitis
- Subarachnoid hemorrhage
- Subdural hematoma
- Trauma
- Tumors

Pre-eclampsia

Psychogenic polydipsia

Pulmonary/chest disorders

- Aspergillosis
- Bronchiectasis
- Bronchogenic carcinoma

- Cystic fibrosis
- Empyema
- Pneumonia (viral and bacterial)
- Positive pressure ventilation
- Tuberculosis

Renal disorders

- Chronic pyelonephritis
- Nephrotic syndrome
- Polycystic kidney
- Renal artery stenosis or occlusion
- Renal failure
- Salt-losing nephropathies

Reset osmostat syndrome

SIADH

Third space losses

- Burns
- Ileus
- Pancreatitis
- Peritonitis

Key Historical Features

✓ Symptoms of hyponatremia (headache, nausea, lethargy, dizziness, confusion, seizure activity, psychosis, coma)

✓ Past medical history

✓ Past surgical history

✓ Psychiatric history

✓ Medications

✓ Drug use

Suggested Work-Up

Serum osmolality	To evaluate euvolemic or hypovolemic patients
Urine osmolality	To evaluate for SIADH
Urinary sodium excretion	To refine the diagnosis in a patient with low plasma osmolality

Serum electrolytes	To evaluate for hyperkalemia or bicarbonate abnormalities
Serum creatinine	To evaluate renal function
TSH	To evaluate for hypothyroidism
Cortisol and ACTH	To evaluate for Addison's disease

Additional Work-Up

| 24-hour urine collection for protein or spot urine protein/creatinine ratio | If nephrotic syndrome is suspected (greater than 3 grams of protein are present in nephrotic syndrome) |
| Serum triglycerides and protein levels | If pseudohyponatremia is suspected |

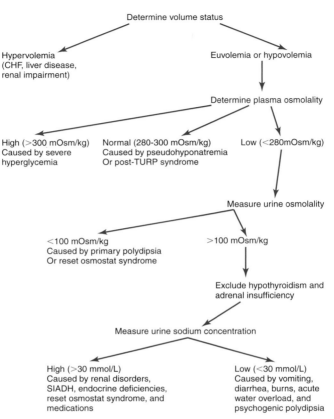

Figure 42-1. Diagnostic algorithm for hyponatremia.

Further reading

Fried LF, Palevsky PM. Hyponatremia and hypernatremia. Medical Clinics of North America 1997;81: 585–609.

Goh KP. Management of hyponatremia. American Family Physician 2004;69: 2387–2394.

Milonis HJ, Liamis GL, Elisaf MS. The hyponatremic patient: a systematic approach to laboratory diagnosis. Canadian Medical Association Journal 2002;166: 1056–1062.

Yeates KE, Singer M, Morton AR. Salt and water: a simple approach to hyponatremia. Canadian Medical Association Journal 2004;170: 365–369.

43 HYPOTHYROIDISM

General Discussion

Hypothyroidism usually results from decreased thyroid hormone production and secretion by the thyroid gland. Hypothyroidism can either be primary or central, which involves the pituitary gland (secondary hypothyroidism) or hypothalamus (tertiary hypothyroidism) and results in a decrease in the release of active TSH. In the United States, the most common cause of hypothyroidism is chronic autoimmune thyroiditis.

Hypothyroidism is far more common in women and in the elderly. In fact, about 2–3% of older women have hypothyroidism. Other risk factors include the presence of thyroid peroxidase antibodies and a high normal level of TSH.

Untreated hypothyroidism can result in decreased cardiac output, memory loss, infertility, and sleep apnea. The American Academy of Family Physicians recommends screening for hypothyroidism in patients 60 years of age or older or those patients with symptoms of hypothyroidism, a family history of thyroid disease, a history of autoimmune disease, or type 1 diabetes.

Myxedema coma refers to severe complications of hypothyroidism, involving hypothermia and stupor or coma. Myxedema coma can be precipitated by mild illnesses, cold exposure, myocardial infarction, and medications that affect the CNS.

Medications That Can Cause Hypothyroidism

Amiodarone

Ethionamide

Interferon alpha

Interleukin-2

Iodine excess

Lithium

Methimazole

Propylthiouracil

Sulfonamides

Causes of Hypothyroidism

Primary hypothyroidism

- Agenesis and dysgenesis of the thyroid
- External irradiation
- Hashimoto's disease (chronic autoimmune thyroiditis)

- Infections
  - Mycobacterium tuberculosis
  - *Pneumocystis carinii*
- Infiltrative disorders
  - Amyloidosis
  - Hemochromatosis
  - Leukemia
  - Lymphoma
  - Sarcoidosis
  - Scleroderma
- Invasive fibrous thyroiditis
- Iodine deficiency
- Medications
- Postpartum thyroiditis
- Radioactive iodine therapy
- Silent thyroiditis
- Subacute thyroiditis
- Thyroid hormone resistance
- Thyroidectomy

Secondary/tertiary hypothyroidism (central hypothyroidism)

- Chronic lymphocytic hypophysitis
- Congenital abnormalities (defects in thyrotropin releasing hormone, TSH, or both)
- Infections
- Infiltrative disorders
- Other brain tumors (nonpituitary)
- Pituitary tumors, metastasis, hemorrhage, necrosis, and aneurysms
- Surgery, trauma

Key Historical Features

✓ Associated symptoms:

- Fatigue
- Weakness
- Depression
- Sleep disturbances
- Decreased appetite
- Memory loss

- Cold intolerance
- Decreased sweating
- Weight gain
- Muscle cramps
- Dry skin
- Brittle nails
- Coarse hair
- Hair loss
- Hearing loss
- Hoarseness
- Swelling of the face
- Pretibial swelling
- Menorrhagia
- Infertility
- Constipation
- Paresthesias
- Changes in taste and smell

✓ Medical history, especially diseases associated with hypothyroidism, such as diabetes mellitus, hyperlipidemia, Sjögren's syndrome, pernicious anemia, systemic lupus erythematous, rheumatoid arthritis, primary biliary cirrhosis, chronic hepatitis, vitiligo, and carpal tunnel syndrome.

Key Physical Findings

✓ Vital signs

✓ Head and neck examination for:

- Thyroid nodules or goiter. Note any thyroidectomy scars
- Ophthalmopathy (proptosis, periorbital edema, conjunctival injection, abnormal extraocular muscle function), which occurs in 4–9% of patients with Hashimoto's thyroiditis
- Pemberton's sign — facial plethora, raised jugular venous pressure (JVP), and inspiratory stridor when the patient raises the arms above her head, indicates a neck mass such as goiter

✓ Cardiovascular examination for

- Bradycardia is associated with hypothyroidism
- Pericardial effusion

✓ Gastrointestinal examination for ascites

✓ Pulmonary examination for a pleural effusion

✓ Neurologic examination for proximal weakness, peripheral neuropathy, and a slow return phase of deep tendon reflexes

Suggested Work-Up

TSH	TSH will be high in primary hypothyroidism and subclinical hypothyroidism and will be low/normal or minimally elevated in central hypothyroidism
Free thyroxine (T4)	Low in primary and central hypothyroidism, normal in subclinical hypothyroidism, high in peripheral thyroid hormone resistance

Additional work-up

Total triiodothyronine (T3)	Less useful than T4 because it may be normal in patients with hypothyroidism
Thyroid peroxidase (TPO) autoantibodies	Often detectable in patients with Hashimoto's thyroiditis (useful in patients with subclinical hypothyroidism)
Thyroglobulin autoantibodies	Usually present with Hashimoto's thyroiditis, although less commonly present than TPO autoantibodies
MRI of the brain and pituitary gland	If central hypothyroidism is present
Thyroid ultrasound	If a thyroid nodule is detected on examination
Fine needle aspiration	To determine if a palpable nodule is malignant
LH, FSH, cortisol level, prolactin, insulin-like growth factor-1 (IGF-1)	If central hypothyroidism is diagnosed (to evaluate for hypopituitarism)
Thyrotropin releasing hormone stimulating test	To distinguish secondary from tertiary hypothyroidism
Electrolytes	Severe hypothyroidism may result in hyponatremia

Lipid panel	Hypothyroidism is associated with elevated triglycerides and elevated low-density lipoprotein cholesterol
Complete blood count	Hypothyroidism is associated with anemia
Fasting blood sugar	To evaluate for diabetes

References

American Association of Clinical Endocrinologists. Medical guidelines for clinical practice for the evaluation and treatment of hyperthyroidism and hypothyroidism. Endocrine Practice 2002;8(6): 458–469.

Devdhar M, Ousman YH, Burman KD. Hypothyroidism. Endocrinology and Metabolism Clinics of North America 2007;36: 595–615.

Hueston WJ. Treatment of hypothyroidism. American Family Physician 2001;64: 1717–1724.

Schmidt DN, Wallace K. How to diagnose hypopituitarism. Postgraduate Medicine 1998;104(7): 77–78, 81–87.

Wartofsky L, Van Nostrand, D. Overt and 'subclinical' hypothyroidism in women. Obstetrical and Gynecological Survey 2006;61(8): 535–542.

General Discussion

Infertility affects one couple in six and becomes more common with increasing age. Clinical evaluation of infertility is indicated if a pregnancy has not occurred after 1 year of regular unprotected intercourse. An infertility work-up should also be initiated on female patients who complain of infertility and have any of the following abnormalities: irregular menses or amenorrhea, bleeding between periods, dyspareunia, history of upper genital tract infection, history of a ruptured appendix or other abdominal surgery, or age greater than 35 years.

Because men account for some 40% of all infertility, the male partner should be evaluated early in the infertility work-up. Historical factors affecting the male partner should also be considered in determining when to begin an infertility evaluation. The following historical factors in the male partner warrant an early investigation: difficulty achieving or maintaining an erection, inability to ejaculate during intercourse, history of testicular injury, history of mumps, history of an undescended testicle, or history of infection in the prostate gland, epididymis, or testicles.

There are several tests that every infertile couple should have performed. The first is a semen analysis of the male partner regardless of how many pregnancies he has caused because sperm counts can change over time. The second test is a hysterosalpingogram (HSG), which helps determine whether the uterine cavity is normal in size and shape and whether the fallopian tubes are patent. Though the HSG is the initial test to evaluate tubal patency, patients at high risk for infection, such as those with a history of clinically diagnosed pelvic inflammatory disease (PID), are best evaluated initially via laparoscopy and hysteroscopy. Laparoscopy is more invasive than HSG, but remains the best test to identify endometriosis and peritubal adhesions.

Routine hormonal assessment, especially in a young apparently ovulatory patient, is controversial. There is less disagreement about performing a hormonal assessment in women aged 35 years and older. The suggested work-up is outlined below.

Approximately 5–10% of infertile couples proceed through a complete infertility evaluation without a cause identified and are said to have unexplained infertility. Additional specialized testing may be performed by infertility clinics, such as ultrasound, antisperm antibodies, and sperm function assays. Empiric treatment regimens have been designed to treat subtle disorders that may not be diagnosed.

Causes of Female Infertility

Endometriosis

Male factors

Ovulatory dysfunction

- Amenorrhea
- Hyperprolactinemia
- Oligomenorrhea

Tubal disease

Uterine causes

- Intrauterine synechiae (Asherman's syndrome)
- Septate uterus
- Uterine fibroids

Unexplained infertility

Key Historical Features

✓ Patient age

✓ Duration of infertility

✓ Timing of sexual intercourse

✓ Galactorrhea

✓ History of dyspareunia

✓ Age at menarche

✓ Intermenstrual bleeding

✓ Determination of whether the woman is currently having regular, monthly menstrual cycles

✓ Prior contraceptive use

✓ Reproductive history, especially previous pregnancies with the same male partner

✓ Medical history, especially thyroid disorders and diabetes mellitus

✓ Surgical history, especially appendectomy or other abdominal surgery

✓ Gynecologic history, especially sexually transmitted diseases, pelvic inflammatory disease, uterine fibroids, pelvic irradiation, or previous use of an intrauterine device

✓ Medications, especially oral contraceptives

✓ Family history, especially genetic diseases

✓   Cigarette smoking

✓   Caffeine use

✓   Alcohol use

✓   Illicit drug use

Key Physical Findings

✓   Height and weight

✓   Skin examination for acne or hirsutism

✓   Pelvic examination for evidence of infection, uterine fibroids, ovarian cysts, or endometriosis

✓   Genital examination of the male partner for phimosis, balanitis, testicular size, or evidence of testicular tumor

Suggested Work-Up

Semen analysis	To evaluate for a male factor for infertility
HSG	To evaluate the uterine cavity and determine whether the fallopian tubes are patent
TSH	To evaluate for thyroid disorders
Prolactin level	To evaluate for hyperprolactinemia
Estradiol and follicle-simulating hormone (FSH) level on cycle day 3	For patients aged 35 years and older to help determine ovarian reserve. Elevated basal FSH levels greater than 8–10 mIU/mL suggest declining fertility potential, and a concentration greater than 20 mIU/mL virtually excludes the chance of a spontaneous pregnancy
Serum progesterone on cycle day 21	A level above 10 ng/mL confirms that ovulation has occurred

Additional Work-Up

Basal body temperature measurement	May be used to help predict the timing of ovulation, but no longer recommended as part of the routine investigation of the infertile couple

Clomiphene citrate challenge test	May be used to increase the sensitivity of a basal FSH determination. The FSH level is measured both before and after the administration of 100 mg of clomiphene citrate during day 5 through day 9 of the menstrual cycle. Elevation in the serum FSH level after the clomiphene citrate challenge indicates decreased ovarian reserve
Total testosterone and dehydroepiandrosterone sulfate levels	If signs of androgen excess are found on physical examination
Laparoscopy	Laparoscopy is generally indicated in women with otherwise unexplained infertility and when there is evidence or suspicion of endometriosis, intrapelvic adhesions, or fallopian tube disease, particularly if the HSG suggests tubal disease that may be amenable to surgical repair
Serum antibody to *Chlamydia trachomatis*	May be used as a screening tool for tubal pathologic conditions in infertile women
Cervical cultures	Routine cervical cultures to identify active current infection with chlamydia or gonorrhea in low-risk populations tends to be unrevealing
Postcoital test	Indirectly measures cervical mucus competency. Postcoital tests are not routinely performed as part of the basic infertility evaluation because of marked variability in performance and variable interpretation
Endometrial biopsy	Provides an indirect measure of ovulation and evaluates the cumulative effect of progesterone on the endometrium. However, there is little role for routine endometrial biopsy as part of a general infertility evaluation
Sonohysterography	May be used as an alternative to HSG to evaluate the uterine cavity but provides little information about the patency of the fallopian tubes

| MRI | May be helpful in visualizing the uterine cavity and determining tubal patency |

References

Brugh VM, Nudell DM, Lipshultz LI. What the urologist should know about the female infertility evaluation. Urology Clinics of North America 2002;29: 983–992.

Hargreave TB, Mills JA. Investigating and managing infertility in general practice. British Medical Journal 1998;316: 1438–1441.

Illions EH, Valley MT, Kaunitz AM. Infertility: a clinical guide for the internist. Medical Clinics of North America 1998;82: 271–295.

Penzias AS. Infertility: contemporary office-based evaluation and treatment. Obstetrics and Gynecology Clinics 2000;27: 473–486.

Smith S, Pfeifer SM, Collins JA. Diagnosis and management of female infertility. Journal of the American Medical Association 2003;290: 1767–1770.

Taylor A. ABC of subfertility: extent of the problem. British Medical Journal 2003;327: 434–436.

45 INFERTILITY, MALE

General Discussion

Infertility, defined as the inability to conceive after 1 year of unprotected intercourse, affects 15% of couples. Half of these couples have a component of male factor infertility, and 20–30% is caused solely by a male factor. The most common male factor is a varicocele. Evaluation of male fertility should be a routine part of the evaluation of an infertile couple, because 50% of male infertility is potentially correctable.

Endocrine disorders remain an important etiology of male infertility and may be associated with significant medical pathology, which may have important implications both for the male and for his potential offspring.

Medications Associated with Male Infertility

Chemotherapy

Cimetidine

Narcotics

Nitrofurantoin

Sulfasalazine

Causes of Male Infertility

Abnormal spermatogenesis

Alcohol abuse

Anabolic steroid use

Androgen resistance

Anorchia

Caffeine excess

Congenital adrenal hyperplasia

Cryptorchidism

Cushing's syndrome

Cystic fibrosis

Diabetes mellitus

Erectile dysfunction

Gonadotoxin exposure (organic solvents, pesticides, excessive heat, heavy metals)

Hypogonadotropic hypogonadism

Marijuana use

Medications/chemotherapy

Multiple sclerosis

Obstruction

Pelvic injury/surgery

Primary hypogonadism

Prolactinoma

Radiation exposure

Sexually transmitted disease

Testicular torsion

Thyroid dysfunction

Tobacco use

Trauma

Tuberculosis

Varicocele

Viral orchitis

Key Historical Features

✓ Duration of the infertility

✓ Previous evaluation and treatment for infertility

✓ Previous pregnancies for either partner

✓ Frequency and timing of intercourse

✓ Sexual dysfunction

✓ Use of lubricants during intercourse

✓ Previous testicular disorders such as cryptorchidism or torsion

✓ Past medical history, especially diabetes or thyroid disorders

✓ Surgical history, especially inguinal, scrotal or retroperitoneal surgery

✓ Family history

✓ Medications

✓ Alcohol

✓ Tobacco use

✓ Caffeine intake

✓ Use of illicit drugs, especially anabolic steroids

✓ History of sexually transmitted disease

✓ Exposure to environmental toxins or radiation exposure

✓ Review of systems

- Anosmia suggests a hypothalamic or pituitary etiology
- Frequent respiratory infections suggests Young's syndrome or Kartagener's syndrome
- Headaches, galactorrhea, and visual field disturbances suggest a CNS tumor

Key Physical Findings

✓   Hair and fat distribution

✓   Examination for gynecomastia

✓   Position and size of the urethral meatus

✓   Testicular size

✓   Presence of varicocele

✓   Presence and contour of vasa differentia and epididymides

✓   Prostate examination

Suggested Work-Up

Semen analysis (2 samples taken 2 weeks apart)	To evaluate semen variables
Serum testosterone	To evaluate for underlying endocrine disorders
FSH	Low level suggests testicular failure
Luteinizing hormone	Low level with low testosterone suggests hypogonadotropic hypogonadism
Prolactin	To evaluate for hyperprolactinemia

Additional Work-Up

Fasting blood glucose	If diabetes mellitus is suspected
TSH	If hypo- or hyperthyroidism is suspected
24-hour urinary free cortisol level	If Cushing's syndrome is suspected
Serum 17-hydroxyprogesterone	If congenital adrenal hyperplasia is suspected

| Quantitation of leukocytes in semen | May help identify underlying infection or inflammation in the semen |
| Antisperm antibody testing | The presence of antisperm antibody correlates with lower pregnancy rates |

References

Brugh VM, Lipshultz LI. Male factor infertility: evaluation and management. Medical Clinics of North America 2004;88: 367–385.

Jarow JP. Endocrine causes of male infertility. Urologic Clinics of North America 2003; 30: 83–90.

Kolettis PN. Evaluation of the subfertile man. American Family Physician 2000;67: 2165–2172.

Spitz A, Kim ED, Lipshultz LI. Contemporary approach to the male infertility evaluation. Obstetrics and Gynecology Clinics 2000;27: 487–516.

General Discussion

Insomnia is a symptom complex consisting of inadequate or poor-quality sleep characterized by one or more of the following problems: difficulty falling asleep, difficulty staying asleep, waking up too early in the morning, and sleep that is not refreshing. Insomnia also involves daytime consequences such as lack of energy, fatigue, irritability, and difficulty concentrating. Acute insomnia represents periods of sleep difficulty lasting between 1 night and a few weeks. Chronic insomnia is sleep difficulty occurring at least 3 nights per week for 1 month or more.

Insomnia is one of the most common concerns encountered in clinical practice though rates of insomnia vary considerably by study. Thirty to 40 percent of adults indicate some level of insomnia within any given year. Insomnia is more common in women and the elderly. Insomnia experienced by older adults is more common in those who have chronic disease and poor health, suggesting that insomnia is not necessarily a direct consequence of aging.

Five major diagnostic categories have been established for chronic insomnia: medical, psychiatric, circadian, pharmacologic, and primary sleep disorder. Primary insomnia is sleeplessness that is not attributable to a medical, psychiatric, or environmental cause.

Most cases of insomnia develop initially in response to a medical or psychosocial stressor. As sleeplessness persists, the patient may begin to associate the bed with wakefulness and heightened arousal rather than sleep, thus perpetuating the insomnia. In general, individuals with prolonged periods of wakefulness before, after, or during sleep are likely to have a behavioral, psychiatric, or circadian disorder. In contrast, patients whose symptoms are primarily frequent, brief nocturnal awakenings, sleep fragmentation, or nonrefreshing sleep are more likely to have a medical or primary sleep disorder.

One model of insomnia conceptualizes predisposing, precipitating, and perpetuating factors. Predisposing factors are those which increase one's vulnerability to insomnia and may include personality characteristics, lifestyle, and extreme circadian rhythm tendencies. A precipitant may be any major stressor such as situational crises and medical, psychiatric, and underlying sleep disorders. Perpetuating factors include maladaptive responses to the initial sleep difficulty such as daytime napping or the use of alcohol to help with sleep.

Medications Associated with Insomnia

Albuterol

Beta blockers

Dextroamphetamine

Diuretics

Methylphenidate

Pemoline

Phenylephrine

Phenylpropanolamine

Pseudoephedrine

Quinidine

Selective serotonin reuptake inhibitors

Steroids

Theophylline

Causes of Insomnia

Caffeine

Dementia

Diet pills

Environmental causes

- Caffeine or alcohol intake before bedtime
- Daytime napping
- Eating or exercising before bedtime
- Noise
- Jet lag
- Shift work
- Temperature issues

Medical conditions

- Alcohol intoxication or withdrawal
- Asthma
- Drug intoxication or withdrawal
- Dyspnea from cardiac or pulmonary disease
- Gastroesophageal reflux disease
- Hormone changes associated with pregnancy, perimenopause, and menopause
- Immobility
- Pain (acute or pain syndromes)
- Thyrotoxicosis

Nicotine

Primary sleep disorders

- Circadian rhythm sleep disorders
- Nocturnal myoclonus
- Obstructive sleep apnea
- Periodic limb movement disorder
- Restless leg syndrome

Psychiatric causes

- Anxiety
- Bedtime worrying
- Conditioning
- Depression
- Hypomania
- Life stressors
- Mania

Key Historical Features

✓ Onset of sleep problems

✓ Recent quality of sleep

✓ Daytime consequences of poor sleep

✓ Difficulty staying awake during tasks, especially driving

✓ Sleep environment, especially noise, light, temperature, and interruptions

✓ Symptoms related to restless leg syndrome such as uncomfortable feelings in the legs which are relieved by moving the legs

✓ Reports by the bed partner of jerking of the arms or legs during sleep

✓ Snoring, gasping, choking, or apneic episodes while sleeping

✓ History of shift work

✓ Hours of work

✓ Bedtime and rise time on weekdays and weekends

✓ Past medical history

✓ Psychiatric history

✓ Medications (prescription and over-the-counter)

✓ Caffeine intake

✓ Alcohol use

✓ Tobacco use

Suggested Work-Up

The evaluation of insomnia is primarily historical, as outlined above.

It often is helpful to ask the patient to keep a sleep diary for a few weeks to record bedtime, total sleep time, time until sleep onset, number of awakenings, use of sleep medications, time out of bed in the morning, a rating of the quality of sleep, and daytime symptoms of sleep deprivation.

TSH	To evaluate for thyrotoxicosis

Additional Work-Up

Polysomnography	To establish the cause when an underlying sleep disorder is suspected by the history

Further reading

American Psychiatric Association Task Force on DSM-IV. Diagnostic and Statistical Manual of Mental Disorders (DSM-IV), 4th ed. Washington, DC: American Psychiatric Association; 1994.

Eddy M, Walbroehl GS. Insomnia. American Family Physician 1999;59: 1911–1916.

National Heart, Lung, and Blood Institute Working Group on Insomnia. Insomnia: assessment and management in primary care. American Family Physician 1999;59: 3029–3038.

Neubauer DN. Insomnia. Primary Care Clinics in Office Practice 2005;32: 375–388.

Roth T, Roehrs T. Insomnia: epidemiology, characteristics, and consequences. Clinical Cornerstone 2003;5: 5–15.

General Discussion

Leukocytosis is defined as a white blood cell (WBC) count greater than 11 000 per mm^3. Circulating leukocytes consist of neutrophils, monocytes, eosinophils, basophils, and lymphocytes. Any one or all of these cell types may increase to abnormal levels in peripheral blood in response to various stimuli. An increase in neutrophils is the most common cause of leukocytosis. In most instances, elevated WBC counts are the result of normal bone marrow reacting to infection or inflammation. Leukocytosis may also occur as a result of physical or emotional stress. Causes of stress leukocytosis include anxiety, overexertion, seizures, anesthesia, and epinephrine administration. Stress leukocytosis reverses within hours of elimination of the causative factor. Leukocytosis may also be caused by medications, malignancy, hemolytic anemia, and splenectomy.

A WBC response of more than 50 000 per mm^3 associated with a cause outside the bone marrow is termed a leukemoid reaction, which is usually caused by a relatively benign process such as infection or inflammation.

Certain clinical factors increase the suspicion that a leukocytosis may be caused by an underlying bone marrow disorder. These factors include a WBC count greater than 30 000 per mm^3, concurrent anemia or thrombocytopenia, life-threatening infection or immunosuppression, lethargy, or significant weight loss. Other concerning factors include bleeding, bruising, or petechiae. Evidence of enlargement of the liver, spleen, or lymph nodes also suggests an underlying bone marrow disorder. The first step in evaluating a leukocytosis is to examine the WBC differential to determine which WBC type is elevated.

Neutrophilia usually reflects the inflammatory response to acute or subacute infections, so it should trigger a diagnostic search for its cause. When neutrophilia occurs in the absence of evidence of acute inflammation or illness, other explanations should be considered. These include chemical effects from medications, malignancies, and chronic myeloproliferative disorders. A peripheral blood smear that shows circulating blasts suggests an acute leukemia and leukoerythroblastic blasts suggests myelofibrosis or another marrow-infiltrating process. In the case of a simple left-shifted neutrophilia, chronic myelogenous leukemia (CML) or another myeloproliferative disorder must be distinguished from a leukemoid reaction. Diagnostic tests are available to help make this distinction and are outlined below.

Monocytosis is defined as absolute peripheral blood monocyte counts greater than 0.50×10^9/L. Monocytosis is often seen in patients with tuberculosis, syphilis, sarcoidosis, fungal infections, and ulcerative colitis. Mild monocytosis is common with Hodgkin's disease and a variety of cancers.

Significant monocytosis is most often seen with hematopoietic malignancies. Monocytosis that persists should be considered a marker of a myeloproliferative disorder until proved otherwise by bone marrow biopsy and cytogenetic studies.

Eosinophilia occurs when the eosinophil count in the peripheral blood exceeds 0.4×10^9/L. The first diagnostic step is to exclude the possibility that eosinophilia is caused by drugs, parasite infection, asthma, allergic conditions, vasculitides, lymphoma, or metastatic cancer.

Peripheral blood basophilia is very rare and suggests chronic basophilic leukemia. Bone marrow biopsy and hematology consultation are recommended.

Lymphocytosis is defined as a lymphocyte count greater than 5.0×10^9/L. Mild to moderate lymphocytosis (lymphocyte counts less than 12×10^9/L) is most commonly caused by viral infection. With the exception of pertussis, acute bacterial infections rarely cause lymphocytosis. Most patients with lymphocytosis have signs of an underlying illness. In patients who do not have evidence of an infectious process or benign disorder, the diagnostic approach depends on establishing a tissue diagnosis to exclude malignant disease.

Causes of Neutrophilia

Chemicals

- Ethylene glycol
- Histamine
- Mercury poisoning
- Venoms (reptiles, insects, jellyfish)

Drugs

- Corticosteroids
- Epinephrine
- Lithium
- Granulocyte colony stimulating factor
- Granulocyte–macrophage colony stimulating factor

Endocrine and metabolic disorders

- Ketoacidosis
- Lactic acidosis
- Thyrotoxicosis

Infections

- Bacteria
- Fungi
- Parasites
- *Rickettsia*
- Viruses

Myeloproliferative disorders
- Acute leukemia
- Agnogenic myeloid metaplasia
- Chronic myelogenous leukemia
- Essential thrombocytosis
- Polycythemia vera

Neoplastic disorders
- Breast carcinoma
- Bronchogenic carcinoma
- Gastric carcinoma
- Lymphoma, especially Hodgkin's disease
- Melanoma
- Metastatic cancer to bone marrow
- Pancreatic carcinoma
- Renal cell carcinoma

Non-neoplastic hematologic disorders
- Acute hemolytic anemias
- Acute transfusion reactions
- Postsplenectomy
- Recovery from marrow failure

Other disorders
- Eclampsia
- Exfoliative dermatitis
- Hypoxia
- Pregnancy
- Tissue necrosis

Rheumatologic and autoimmune disorders
- Autoimmune hemolytic anemia
- Gout
- Inflammatory bowel disease
- Rheumatoid arthritis
- Vasculitis

Trauma
- Crush injury
- Electrical injury
- Hypothermia
- Thermal injury

Causes of Eosinophilia

Adrenal insufficiency

Allergic reactions

Dermatologic conditions

Hyper-eosinophilic syndrome

Immunologic disorders

- Eosinophilia–myalgia syndrome
- Lupus erythematosus
- Periarteritis
- Rheumatoid arthritis

Infections

- Chorea
- Genitourinary infections
- Leprosy
- Parasitic infections
- Scarlet fever

Malignancy

- Hodgkin's lymphoma
- Non-Hodgkin's lymphoma

Myeloproliferative disorders

- Chronic myelogenous leukemia
- Myelofibrosis
- Polycythemia vera

Pleural and pulmonary conditions

- Loffler's syndrome
- Pulmonary infiltrates

Sarcoidosis

Causes of Basophilia

Alteration of marrow and reticuloendothelial compartments

- Chronic hemolytic anemia
- Hodgkin's disease
- Splenectomy

Endocrine causes

- Estrogens
- Hypothyroidism
- Ovulation

Infections

- Chronic sinusitis
- Viral infections (varicella)

Inflammatory conditions

- Chronic airway inflammation
- Chronic dermatitis
- Inflammatory bowel disease

Myeloproliferative disorders

- Chronic myelogenous leukemia
- Myelofibrosis
- Polycythemia vera

Causes of Lymphocytosis

Acute infections

- Acute infectious lymphocytosis
- Adenovirus
- Brucellosis
- Coxsackie virus
- Cytomegalo virus infection
- Epstein–Barr virus infection
- Hepatitis
- HIV infection
- Measles
- Mumps
- Pertussis
- Syphilis (secondary)
- Toxoplasmosis
- Tuberculosis
- Typhoid fever
- Varicella
- Viral infections

Chronic infections

- Brucellosis
- Tuberculosis

Neoplastic disorders

- Acute lymphocytic leukemia
- Carcinoma
- Chronic lymphocytic leukemia
- Chronic myelogenous leukemia

- Hodgkin's disease
- Thymoma

Other conditions

- Drug reactions
- Graves' disease
- Sjögren's syndrome

Causes of Monocytosis

Gastrointestinal disorders

- Cirrhosis
- Granulomatous colitis
- Ulcerative colitis

Infections

- Brucellosis
- Endocarditis
- Fungal infections
- Paratyphoid
- Protozoal infections
- Recovery from acute infections
- Syphilis
- Tuberculosis
- Typhoid
- Viral infections (varicella)

Neoplastic diseases

- Acute monocytic leukemia
- Acute myelomonocytic leukemia
- Chronic lymphocytic leukemia
- Chronic myelomonocytic leukemia
- Carcinoma
- Hodgkin's disease
- Juvenile chronic myelomonocytic leukemia
- Multiple myeloma
- Myelodysplasia
- Waldenstrom's macroglobulinemia

Other disorders

- Congenital neutropenia
- Drug reactions
- Recovery from marrow suppression
- Sarcoidosis

Key Historical Features

✓ Fever

✓ Sweats

✓ Weight loss

✓ Easy bruising or bleeding

✓ Past medical history

✓ Medications

Key Physical Findings

✓ Vital signs for evidence of fever

✓ Pallor

✓ Evidence of lymphadenopathy

✓ Abdominal examination for hepatomegaly or splenomegaly

✓ Skin and extremity examination for purpura or petechiae

Suggested Work-Up of Leukocytosis

WBC with differential	To determine which WBC type is elevated
Peripheral blood smear	To exclude the possibility of an acute leukemia and to classify the process as granulocytosis (neutrophilia, eosinophilia, or basophilia), monocytosis, or lymphocytosis

Suggested Work-Up of Neutrophilia

Leukocyte alkaline phosphatase (LAP)	LAP usually increased when neutrophilia represents a reaction to an acute illness. LAP score is markedly decreased in cases of chronic myelogenous leukemia
Peripheral blood FISH for *bcr/abl*	To evaluate for CML if the patient's history does not suggest a leukemoid reaction
Hematology consultation and bone marrow aspiration	May be required to help determine the cause of neutrophilia

Suggested Work-Up of Monocytosis

Monocytosis that persists or does not obviously accompany a chronic infectious, inflammatory, or granulomatous process warrants hematology consultation.

Suggested Work-Up of Eosinophilia

Stool test for ova and parasites	To evaluate for gastrointestinal parasitic infection

For primary eosinophilia (not due to drugs, parasitic infection, asthma, allergic conditions, etc.), the following tests are suggested:

Serum tryptase	Increased levels suggest mastocytosis
T-cell immunophenotyping and TCR gene rearrangement analysis	Positive test results suggest an underlying clonal T-cell disorder
Serum interleukin 5	Elevated level requires evaluation of the bone marrow for the presence of a clonal T-cell disease
Serum IgE level	Increased IgE level may decrease the risk of developing eosinophilia-associated heart disease
Bone marrow biopsy, including cytogenetic studies, FISH for FIP1L1-PDGFRA mutation, immunohistochemical stains for tryptase, and mast cell immunophenotyping	Recommended in all patients with primary eosinophilia to distinguish between clonal eosinophilia and the hyper-eosinophilic syndrome

Suggested Work-Up of Basophilia

Bone marrow biopsy and hematology consultation	To evaluate for chronic basophilic leukemia

Suggested Work-Up of Lymphocytosis

Bone marrow biopsy	Required when the peripheral blood smear shows leukoerythroblastosis or lymphoblasts. Also required if the lymphocytosis persists in a patient who has no evidence of acute or subacute infection

| Immunophenotyping by flow cytometry | To provide evidence for or against dominance of one lymphocyte type and differentiation stage |
| Hematology consultation | Recommended for any lymphocytosis that is not reactive |

References

Abramson N, Melton B. Leukocytosis: basics of clinical assessment. American Family Physician 2000;62: 2053–2060.

Bagby GC. Leukopenia and leukocytosis. In: Goldman L, ed. Cecil textbook of medicine, 22nd ed. Philadelphia: Saunders; 2004.

Tefferi A, Hanson CA, Inwards DJ. How to interpret and pursue an abnormal complete blood cell count in adults. Mayo Clinic Proceedings 2005;80: 923–936.

General Discussion

The normal peripheral white blood cell count ranges from 5.0 to 10.0×10^9/L. Leukopenia is defined as a total WBC count below 4.5×10^9/L. When leukopenia is discovered, the first step is to determine which type of WBC is at lower levels than normal.

Neutropenia occurs when a patient's peripheral neutrophil count is less than 2.0×10^9/L. The normal range in Yemenite Jews and African Americans is somewhat lower, and neutropenia is defined as counts less than 1.5×10^9/L in these populations. The risk of bacterial infection is substantially increased when the peripheral neutrophil count falls below 0.5×10^9/L. The diagnostic evaluation of neutropenia must first address whether the patient has fever, sepsis, or both.

The most frequent cause of acquired neutropenia is medication. Any drug should be considered to be a potential cause until proved otherwise. Neutropenia may also occur as a manifestation of a wide variety of systemic diseases. Infection is a common cause of neutropenia, particularly viral infections and sepsis.

Normal lymphocyte counts range from 2 to 4×10^9/L, with approximately 20% B lymphocytes and 70% T lymphocytes. Lymphocytopenia is defined as a peripheral blood lymphocyte count below 1.5×10^9/L. Protein-calorie malnutrition is the most common cause of lymphocytopenia worldwide. There generally are no specific clinical manifestations of lymphocytopenia. However, the patient may exhibit signs of immunologic deficiency depending upon the underlying cause of the lymphocytopenia, the degree of immunodeficiency, and the duration of the disease.

Medications Associated with Neutropenia

Acetazolamide

Alkylating agents

Allopurinol

Aminopyrine

Anthracyclines

Brompheniramine

Captopril

Carbamazepine

Chloramphenicol

Chlorpromazine

Chlorpropamide

Chlorthalidone

Cimetidine

Cisplatin

Clozapine

Dactinomycin

Dapsone

Ethosuximide

Ganciclovir

Gold salts

Hydrochlorothiazide

Hydroxyurea

Ibuprofen

Indomethacin

Isoniazid

Levamisole

Mephenytoin

Methimazole

Methyldopa

Nitrofurantoin

Para-aminosalicylic acid

Penicillamine

Penicillins

Phenylbutazone

Phenytoin

Procainamide

Prochlorperazine

Promazine

Propranolol

Propylthiouracil

Pyrimethamine

Quinidine

Quinine

Recombinant interferons

Rifampin

Streptokinase

Sulfonamides

Thiouracil

Tocainide

Tolbutamide

Trimethadione

Tripelennamine

Vancomycin

Vinca alkaloids

Zidovudine

Medications Associated with Lymphocytopenia

Cyclophosphamide

Cyclosporine

Cytotoxic chemotherapy

Fludarabine

Glucocorticosteroids

Quinine

Causes of Neutropenia

Acquired aplastic anemia

Benzene toxicity

Congenital neutropenias (Kostmann's syndrome and cyclic neutropenia)

Ethanol

Folate deficiency

Immune-mediated leukopenia

Large granular lymphocyte leukemia

Medications

Metastatic cancer (lung, breast, prostate, stomach, hematopoietic)

Myelodysplastic syndrome

Nonlymphocytic leukemia

Paroxysmal nocturnal hemoglobinuria

Pseudoneutropenia

Sepsis

Viral infections

Vitamin B_{12} deficiency

Causes of Lymphocytopenia

Alcohol abuse

Autoimmune and connective tissue diseases (lupus and rheumatoid arthritis)

Bacterial infections

Chronic renal failure

Chronic right ventricular failure

Congenital immunodeficiency states

- Adenosine deaminase deficiency
- Bruton X-linked agammaglobulinemia
- DiGeorge's syndrome
- Nezelof's syndrome
- Severe combined immunodeficiency
- Wiskott–Aldrich syndrome

Extracorporeal circulation

Graft-versus-host disease

Hemorrhage

Hodgkin's disease

Malnutrition

Medications

Multiple myeloma

Older age

Protein-losing enteropathy

Radiation

Sarcoidosis

Sepsis

Severe acute respiratory syndrome

Surgery

Thoracic duct drainage or rupture

Thymoma

Trauma

Tuberculosis or other granulomatous infection

Viral infections, especially AIDS

Key Historical Features

✓   Attempt to determine the chronicity of the neutropenia

✓   Fever

✓   Symptoms of underlying systemic disease

✓   Past medical history

✓   Medications

Key Physical Findings

✓   Vital signs, especially presence of fever

✓   Thorough examination for a source of infection, with special attention to the lungs, genitourinary system, gastrointestinal system, oropharynx, and skin

Suggested Work-Up of Neutropenia

Examination of the peripheral blood smear and differential WBC count	To determine the WBC line involved
Lymphocyte immunophenotyping by flow cytometry	To evaluate for leukemia
T-cell receptor gene rearrangement studies	To evaluate for leukemia
Antineutrophil antibody testing	To evaluate for immune-mediated disease

Suggested Work-Up of Lymphocytopenia

Quantification of B cells, CD4+, and CD8+	To evaluate the subsets of lymphocytes remaining in the circulation
Quantitative immunoglobulin levels	To detect deficiencies of cell-mediated immunity

Additional Work-Up

Serum folate, homocysteine, methylmalonic acid, and vitamin B_{12} levels	If folate or vitamin B_{12} deficiency is suspected

References

Bagby GC. Leukopenia and leukocytosis. In: Goldman L, ed. Cecil textbook of medicine, 22nd ed. Philadelphia: Saunders; 2004.

Tefferi A, Hanson CA, Inwards DJ. How to interpret and pursue an abnormal complete blood cell count in adults. Mayo Clinic Proceedings 2005;80: 923–936.

General Discussion

The first step in the evaluation of muscle weakness is differentiating true muscle weakness from fatigue and asthenia. Fatigue is the inability to continue performing a task after multiple repetitions while asthenia is a sense of exhaustion in the absence of actual muscle weakness.

Peripheral nerve lesions must be distinguished from CNS disease. Peripheral neuropathies and myopathies usually follow a gradual progressive deterioration while central lesions are more commonly acute or subacute.

The history and physical examination represent an important part of the evaluation of muscle weakness. Details of the history and physical examination are outlined below. Disease onset and progression as well as the pattern of muscle weakness are key historical features. During the physical examination, the muscle weakness must be objectively confirmed, quantified, and localized if possible.

The laboratory and radiographic evaluation should be guided by findings from the history and physical examination. In the absence of features suggesting a particular diagnosis, the evaluation may proceed in a stepwise fashion, beginning with a general laboratory evaluation as outlined below.

Medications Associated with Muscle Weakness

Amiodarone

Chemotherapeutic agents

Cimetidine

Corticosteroids

Gemfibrozil

Interferon

Lamivudine

Leuprolide acetate

Methimazole

NSAIDs

Penicillin

Propylthiouracil

Statins (HMG-CoA reductase inhibitors)

Sulfonamides

Zidovudine

Causes of Muscle Weakness

Cocaine use

Electrolyte imbalance

- Hypercalcemia
- Hyperkalemia
- Hypermagnesemia
- Hypokalemia
- Hypomagnesemia

Endocrine causes

- Acromegaly
- Hyperparathyroidism
- Hyperthyroidism
- Hypopituitarism
- Hypothyroidism
- Vitamin D deficiency

Genetic causes

- Distal myopathies
- Muscular dystrophy
- Myotonic dystrophy type 2

Infectious causes

- Diphtheria
- Epstein–Barr virus
- HIV
- Influenza
- Lyme disease
- Meningitis
- Polio
- Rabies
- Syphilis
- Tetanus
- Tick paralysis
- Toxoplasmosis

Metabolic causes

- Acid maltase deficiency
- Aldolase A deficiency
- Brancher enzyme deficiency
- Carnitine deficiency
- Carnitine palmitoyltransferase II deficiency

- Myophosphorylase deficiency
- Phosphofructokinase deficiency
- Mitochondrial defects
- Trifunctional protein deficiency

Neurologic causes

- Amyotrophic lateral sclerosis
- Botulism
- Carbamate intoxication
- Cerebrovascular accident
- Cervical spondylosis
- Degenerative disk disease
- Epidural hematoma
- Guillain–Barré syndrome
- Lambert-Eton myasthenic syndrome
- Multiple sclerosis
- Myasthenia gravis
- Neoplasm
- Organophosphate intoxication
- Spinal cord injury
- Spinal muscle atrophy
- Subdural hematoma

Rheumatologic causes

- Dermatomyositis
- Inclusion body myositis
- Polymyalgia rheumatica
- Polymyositis
- Rheumatoid arthritis
- Systemic lupus erythematosus
- Systemic sclerosis/scleroderma

Other causes

- Alcohol toxicity
- Amyloidosis
- Sarcoidosis

Key Historical Features

✓ Age
✓ Onset of symptoms
✓ Rate of progression of symptoms

- ✓ Pattern of muscle weakness
    - Global or focal
    - Proximal or distal
    - Unilateral or bilateral
- ✓ Associated symptoms
    - Abdominal pain
    - Arthralgias
    - Constipation
    - Diarrhea
    - Dysphagia
    - Easy bruising
    - Malaise
    - Menorrhagia
    - Rash
    - Weakness associated with exercise or activity
- ✓ Past medical history
- ✓ Medications
- ✓ Family history
- ✓ Social history
    - Alcohol consumption
    - Drug use
    - Toxin exposure

Key Physical Findings

- ✓ Examination of the thyroid gland
- ✓ Head and neck examination for ptosis or fatigable weakness
- ✓ Assessment of muscle strength
- ✓ Evaluation of ability to stand and write
- ✓ Neurologic examination
- ✓ Mental status testing
- ✓ Cardiac examination
- ✓ Pulmonary examination
- ✓ Skin examination for rash
- ✓ Extremity examination for joint inflammation

Suggested Work-Up

CBC	To evaluate for infection
Electrolytes	To evaluate for potassium imbalance
BUN and creatinine	To evaluate for uremia
Glucose	To evaluate for hypoglycemia or hyperglycemia
Calcium	To evaluate for hypercalcemia
Magnesium	To evaluate for magnesium disorder
Phosphorus	To evaluate for hypophosphatemia
TSH	To evaluate for thyroid-related myopathy
Creatine kinase	May be elevated in inflammatory myopathies, muscular dystrophies, sarcoidosis, alcoholism, infections, storage myopathies, and adverse drug reactions
ESR and ANA	To evaluate for rheumatologic myopathies
Electromyelogram	To help establish the presence of a myopathy and indicate if a neuropathy or neuromuscular disease is present

Additional Work-Up

Brain CT scan or MRI	If cerebrovascular disease is suspected
Lumbar puncture	If meningitis, encephalitis, or multiple sclerosis is suspected
Parathyroid hormone	If hypercalcemia or uremia is present on initial screening
Rheumatoid factor	If rheumatoid arthritis is suspected
Anti-double-stranded DNA, antiphospholipid antibodies, C3 and C4 levels	If lupus is suspected

Anticentromere antibodies	If scleroderma is suspected
AST, ALT, GGT, and vitamin B_{12} level	If alcoholism is suspected
ACTH assay or ACTH stimulation test	If adrenal insufficiency is suspected (hypoglycemia, hyponatremia, hyperkalemia)
24-hour urine cortisol or dexamethasone suppression test	If Cushing's disease is suspected
Growth hormone assay	If acromegaly is suspected
Vitamin D assay	If osteomalacia is suspected
Toxicologic analysis	If toxin exposure is suspected
Pulmonary function tests	If Guillain–Barré syndrome is suspected
Muscle biopsy	If the diagnosis is inconclusive after a thorough history, physical examination, laboratory, radiologic, and electromyographic evaluation

Further reading

Anagnos A, Ruff RL, Kaminski HJ. Endocrine neuromyopathies. Neurologic Clinics 1997; 15: 673–696.

LoVecchio F. Approach to generalized weakness and peripheral neuromuscular disease. Emergency Medicine Clinics of North America 1997;15: 605–623.

O'Rourke KS. Myopathies in the elderly. Rheumatic Diseases Clinics of North America 2000;26: 647–672.

Saguil A. Evaluation of the patient with muscle weakness. American Family Physician 2005; 71: 1327–1336.

Yazici Y, Kagen LJ. Clinical presentation of the idiopathic inflammatory myopathies. Rheumatic Diseases Clinics of North America 2002;28: 823–832.

50 MYALGIAS

General Discussion

Muscle pain may be the result of muscle disease, but joint and bone disease also may produce complaints of muscle pain. Pain from disease of overlying tissue, fascia, or tendons also may be referred to muscle. In addition, disease of major peripheral nerves or of their smaller intramuscular branches may produce both muscle pain and muscle weakness. Muscle pain may be a major symptom in inflammatory, metabolic, endocrine, and toxic myopathies.

Metabolic myopathies is a term applied to a heterogeneous group of disorders that result from the inability of skeletal muscle to produce or maintain adequate levels of energy in the form of adenosyl triphosphate (ATP). The metabolic myopathies are classified according to the altered area of metabolism as muscle glycogenoses, disorders of lipid metabolism, and mitochondrial myopathies. The symptoms of patients with the metabolic myopathies vary widely but include premature fatigue, episodic aches, cramps and pains occasionally accompanied by extensive rhabdomyolysis with myoglobinuria, and fixed, progressive muscle weakness. The diagnosis of a metabolic myopathy usually requires muscle biopsy with a combination of analyses, including histology, histochemistry, electron microscopy, and biochemistry.

Multiple drugs and toxins can cause myopathy. Patients at risk for developing adverse reactions typically are those who have reduced abilities to metabolize or excrete the drug and its metabolites, which include infants, children, elderly patients, and those who have liver or renal failure. There are several recognized mechanisms whereby toxins can produce muscle damage. Toxins may cause a direct toxic or biochemical effect. Secondary effects of toxins resulting in muscle damage include immune activation with inflammation, vascular insufficiency, ischemia, hypokalemia, muscle overactivity, compression, or direct injury resulting from repeated injections. Since toxin-related muscle damage can be readily reversible once exposure stops, toxic myopathies should be considered early in the differential diagnosis of myalgias.

The idiopathic inflammatory myopathies are a group of disorders characterized by proximal muscle weakness and nonsuppurative inflammation of skeletal muscle, often accompanied by extramuscular manifestations. Dermatomyositis, polymyositis, inclusion body myositis, and cancer-associated myositis are idiopathic inflammatory myopathies. Patients with idiopathic inflammatory myopathy may present with a variety of nonspecific symptoms such as fatigue, myalgias, arthralgias, malaise, and weight loss.

Medications Associated with Myalgias

Albuterol

Amiodarone

Amphotericin B

Chloroquine

Cimetidine

Clofibrate

Corticosteroids (chronic use)

Cyclosporine

Diuretics

L-Dopa

Emetine

Enalapril

Epsilon-aminocaproic acid

Finasteride

Gemfibrozil

Halothane

HMG-CoA reductase inhibitors (statins)

Hydroxychloroquine

Interferon-alfa

Isoretinoin

Lamotrigine

Labetalol

Levodopa

Leuprolide

Lovastatin

Meperidine

Nicotinic acid

Omeprazole

Pancuronium

D-Penicillamine

Phenytoin

Pravastatin

Procainamide

Propofol

Quinacrine

Simvastatin

Succinylcholine

Tacrolimus

Tretinoin

L-Tryptophan

Valproic acid

Vincristine

Vitamin E

Zidovudine

Causes of Myalgias

Adrenal insufficiency

Alcohol abuse

Amphetamines

Amyopathic dermatomyositis

Antisynthetase syndrome

Cancer-associated myositis

Cocaine

Dermatomyositis

Disorders of lipid metabolism

Fibromyalgia

Heroin

Infections

- Coxsackie virus
- Influenza virus

Laxatives

Licorice

Medications

Mitochondrial myopathies

Mixed connective tissue syndrome

Muscle glycogenoses

Osteomalacia

Overlap syndromes

Partial defects in dystrophin

Polyarteritis nodosa

Polymyalgia rheumatica

Polymyositis

Rheumatoid arthritis

Scleroderma

Sepsis

Systemic lupus erythematosus

Toluene abuse

Vigorous activity

Key Historical Features

✓ Age of onset

✓ Muscle weakness

✓ Fatigue

✓ Insomnia

✓ Depressive symptoms

✓ Stiffness and pain in the hips and shoulders

✓ Joint pain

✓ Past medical history

✓ Medications

✓ Alcohol use

✓ Substance abuse

✓ Review of systems

Key Physical Findings

✓ Vital signs

✓ Cardiac examination for the presence of cardiomyopathy

✓ Examination of the joints for swelling

✓ Examination of the skin for any skin changes such as rash

✓ Evaluation of muscle strength and identification of the pattern of muscle groups affected

✓ Neurologic examination to screen for the presence of neuropathy

Suggested Work-Up

Serum creatine kinase	To evaluate for muscle fiber necrosis
Urine myoglobin	Nonspecific marker of myopathy. Myoglobin is not normally detectable in urine and myoglobinuria should be suspected when a urine sample tests positive for hemoglobin but urine microscopy reveals no red blood cells

| Electromyography (EMG) | Histologic evaluation may be used to provide information about the extent of myofiber necrosis, the fiber type that is primarily affected, and the presence of vacuoles or inflammation |
| Muscle biopsy | May be needed to confirm the diagnosis and determine the cause of the muscle dysfunction |

Additional Work-Up

ESR	To evaluate for inflammation in polymyalgia rheumatica, temporal arteritis, and other rheumatologic and inflammatory conditions
MRI	May be used as a noninvasive differential diagnostic method
Serum lactic dehydrogenase, aspartate aminotransferase (AST), creatine kinase, and aldolase	If steroid-induced myopathy is suspected
ACTH stimulation test	If adrenal insufficiency is suspected

Further reading

Anagnos A, Ruff RL, Kaminski HJ. Endocrine neuromyopathies. Neurologic Clinics 1997; 15: 673–696.

O'Rourke KS. Myopathies in the elderly. Rheumatic Diseases Clinics of North America 2000;26: 647–672.

Wald JJ. The effects of toxins on muscle. Neurologic Clinics 2000;18(3): 695–718.

Walsh RJ, Amato AA. Toxic myopathies. Neurology Clinics 2005;23: 397–428.

Wortmann RL, DiMauro S. Differentiating idiopathic inflammatory myopathies from metabolic myopathies. Rheumatic Diseases Clinics of North America 2002;28(4): 759–778.

Yazici Y, Kagen LJ. Clinical presentation of the idiopathic inflammatory myopathies. Rheumatic Diseases Clinics of North America 2002;28: 823–832.

51 NEPHROLITHIASIS

General Discussion

The lifetime risk of passing a kidney stone is about 8–10% among North American males, with a peak incidence at age 30 years. Women have a risk about half that of men. Among patients who have passed one kidney stone, the lifetime recurrence rate is 60–80%.

About 80% of kidney stones contain calcium, and the majority of these stones are composed of calcium oxalate. A minority contain calcium phosphate or admixtures of oxalate and phosphate salts. About 10% of stones are composed of uric acid. Another 10% are struvite stones which develop exclusively in patients with urinary tract infections caused by urease-producing organisms such as *Proteus* species. Cystine accounts for about 1% of all stones, but only occur in patients with cystinuria, an autosomal recessive disorder.

Some controversy exists about the extent of investigation required after the passage of a single stone. Since the rate of recurrence is high, many experts favor a thorough evaluation for anyone who has passed a stone. A comprehensive urinary evaluation or referral is required for patients in whom multiple stones are detected clinically or radiographically, patients with anatomic abnormalities of the urinary tract, patients with a strong family history of nephrolithiasis, and patients with cystine or uric acid stones.

Plain abdominal radiography, ultrasonography, intravenous pyelography (IVP), helical CT scanning, and MRI scanning can be used to demonstrate stones in the renal tract. IVP has been considered the gold standard for many years, but noncontrast helical CT scanning is now the preferred imaging modality in many centers because it is faster and more sensitive than IVP and does not require the use of intravenous contrast material. In addition, CT scanning may identify other causes of abdominal pain masquerading as renal colic.

Medications Associated with Nephrolithiasis

Acetazolamide

Ascorbic acid

Calcium supplementation

Carbonic anhydrase inhibitors

Corticosteroids

Cytotoxic agents used for malignancies

Indinavir

Silicate

Sulfonamides

Triamterene

Causes of Nephrolithiasis

Hypercalciuria

Hyperoxaluria

Hyperuricosuria

Hypocitraturia

Idiopathic

Infection (*Proteus, Klebsiella, Serratia*, and *Mycoplasma* urinary tract infection)

Renal tubular acidosis type I

Key Historical Features

✓   Patient age

✓   Frequency of stone formation

✓   Past medical history

- Anatomic abnormalities of the renal system
- Crohn's disease
- Cystinuria
- Gout
- Hypercalciuria
- Hyperoxaluria
- Hyperparathyroidism
- Hyperthyroidism
- Hypocitraturia
- Immobilization
- Immunocompromised status
- Lesch–Nyhan syndrome
- Malignancy
- Milk alkali syndrome
- Polycystic kidney disease
- Recurrent or chronic urinary tract infections
- Renal tubular acidosis
- Sarcoidosis
- Skeletal disease
- Solitary functioning kidney

✓ Past surgical history
- Renal transplant
- Small bowel resection

✓ Medications

✓ Family history
- Stone disease
- Parathyroid disease
- Gout

✓ Occupational history, especially significant sweating

✓ Alcohol use

✓ Dietary history
- Fluid intake
- Calcium intake
- Excessive intake of protein-rich foods
- Excessive intake of chocolate or nuts
- Sodium intake

Key Physical Findings

✓ Vital signs

✓ General examination for diaphoresis or ill appearance

✓ Cardiac examination for tachycardia

✓ Pulmonary examination for tachypnea

✓ Abdominal examination for tenderness, bruits, pulsatile masses, and symmetry of femoral pulses

✓ The bladder should be examined for tenderness and evidence of retention. There should be no peritoneal signs in nephrolithiasis

✓ Back examination for flank or costovertebral angle tenderness

✓ Genitourinary and rectal examinations should be unremarkable in nephrolithiasis

Suggested Work-Up of a Patient with First Stone Episode

Serum electrolytes	Used to calculate the anion gap. Type I renal tubular acidosis presents with a nonanion gap acidosis with concomitant hypokalemia
Blood urea nitrogen and creatinine	To evaluate renal function

Serum calcium	To evaluate for hypercalcemia and hyperparathyroidism
Serum phosphorus	To evaluate for hypophosphatemia
Serum uric acid	To evaluate for hyperuricemia
Pregnancy test	To rule out pregnancy
Urinalysis	Hematuria is present in 90% of patients with stones
	Urinalysis may reveal the presence of a UTI
	Hexagonal crystals suggest cystinuria
	Low urinary pH is associated with uric acid stone formation
	High urinary pH may suggest a struvite stone
	High urinary pH accompanied by a low serum bicarbonate concentration may occur with type I renal tubular acidosis
Urine culture	If urinary infection is suspected
CBC	If infection is suspected
Stone analysis	If the stone is available
Imaging study with ultrasonography, helical CT, or IVP (helical CT generally preferred)	To evaluate for additional stones, radiolucent stones, or anatomic abnormalities
Serum bicarbonate	If type I renal tubular acidosis is suspected

Suggested Work-Up of a Patient with Recurrent Stone Formation

| 24-hour urine collection for: | Used for initial management and to guide therapy. May need to be repeated to monitor effectiveness of treatment |

volume

pH

calcium

phosphate

sodium

uric acid

oxalate

citrate

creatinine

Further reading

Bushinsky DA. Nephrolithiasis. Journal of the American Society of Nephrology 1998;9: 917–924.

Goldfarb DS, Coe FL. Prevention of recurrent nephrolithiasis. American Family Physician 1999;60: 2269–2276.

Manthey DE, Teichman J. Nephrolithiasis. Emergency Medicine Clinics of North America 2001;19: 633–654.

Morton AR, Iliescu EA, Wilson JWL. Nephrology: investigation and treatment of recurrent kidney stones. Canadian Medical Association Journal 2002;166: 213–218.

Tiselius HG. Medical evaluation of nephrolithiasis. Endocrinology and Metabolism Clinics of North America 2002;31: 1031–1050.

52 OSTEOPOROSIS

General Discussion

Primary osteoporosis results from deterioration of bone mass that is related to aging and decreased gonadal function but is not associated with any chronic illness. Because primary osteoporosis results from decreased gonadal function, early menopause or premenopausal estrogen deficiency may hasten the development of osteoporosis. Other risk factors for primary osteoporosis include female gender, white or Asian ancestry, sedentary lifestyle, tobacco use, low calcium intake, and low body weight.

Secondary osteoporosis results from chronic conditions that contribute to accelerated bone density loss. Chronic conditions that may contribute to secondary osteoporosis include acromegaly, alcoholism, anorexia nervosa, chronic liver disease, diabetes mellitus type I, glycogen storage diseases, hemochromatosis, homocystinuria, hyperadrenocorticism, hyperparathyroidism, hyperprolactinemia, hypophosphatasia, malabsorption syndromes and gastric operations, Marfan syndrome, osteogenesis imperfecta, renal disease, thyrotoxicosis, and vitamin D deficiency.

Long-term glucocorticoid therapy is a common cause of osteoporosis. A list of medications that may cause osteoporosis is listed below.

Men are more likely than women to have a secondary cause of osteoporosis. In the patient with osteoporosis, initial evaluation should begin with a risk factor assessment (see risk factors below) and a history and physical examination focusing on signs of chronic disease. If secondary osteoporosis is suspected based upon findings from the history and physical examination, a work-up should be performed.

Medications Associated with Osteoporosis

Cyclosporine

Furosemide

Glucocorticoids

GnRH agonists

Heparin (prolonged treatment)

Methotrexate

Phenobarbital

Phenothiazines

Phenytoin

Thyroid hormone excess

Risk Factors for Osteoporosis

Advancing age

Alcohol abuse

Caucasian or Asian race

Chronic kidney disease

Early menopause

Family history of osteoporosis

Female gender

High caffeine intake

Impaired calcium absorption

Late menarche

Low intake of calcium, phosphorus, or vitamin D

Nulliparity

Low body weight or petite body frame

Sedentary lifestyle

Tobacco use

Suggested Work-Up for Patients with Suspected Secondary Osteoporosis

Serum creatinine	To evaluate for renal disease
ALT and AST	To evaluate for liver disease
Alkaline phosphatase	To evaluate for liver disease, Paget's disease or other bone pathology
Albumin	Decreased levels suggest malnutrition
Serum calcium	Decreased level may indicate malabsorption or vitamin D deficiency
	Increased level may indicate primary hyperparathyroidism or malignancy
Serum iron and ferritin	Levels are increased with hemochromatosis
Serum phosphorus	Decreased level may indicate osteomalacia
TSH	To evaluate for hyperthyroidism
Serum protein electrophoresis, ESR, CBC, serum calcium, parathyroid hormone	Abnormal SPEP, elevated ESR, anemia, hypercalcemia, and depressed PTH suggest multiple myeloma

Testosterone (males)   Decreased levels suggest hypogonadism

Estrogen (females)   Decreased levels in premenopausal women
suggest hypogonadism

1,25 hydroxyvitamin D   Elevated levels occur with 25-hydroxycalciferol
hyperparathyroidism

Decreased levels suggest vitamin D deficiency

24-hour urine calcium   Decreased urinary calcium excretion suggests
measurement   malabsorption or vitamin D deficiency

Additional Work-Up

Dexamethasone   May be indicated when Cushing's syndrome is
suppression test   suspected

Stool for fat or xylose   Used when there is a history of gastrectomy
breath test   or diarrhea to rule out malabsorption

Further reading

Harper KD, Weber TJ. Secondary osteoporosis. Diagnostic considerations. Endocrinology and
Metabolism Clinics of North Am 1998;27(2): 325–348.

Kenny AM, Prestwood KM. Osteoporosis: Pathogenesis, diagnosis, and treatment in older
adults. Rheumatic Diseases Clinics of North America 2000;26: 569–591.

Simon LS. Osteoporosis. Clinics in Geriatric Medicine 2005;21: 603–629.

South-Paul, JE. Osteoporosis: part I: evaluation and assessment. American Family Physician
2001;63: 897–904.

Tresolini CP, Gold DT, Lee LS, eds. Working with patients to prevent, treat and manage
osteoporosis: a curriculum guide for health professions, 2nd ed. San Francisco:
National Fund for Medical Education; 1998.

53 PERIPHERAL EDEMA

General Discussion

Edema results from an imbalance of forces controlling fluid exchange. These forces include increased capillary hydraulic pressure, decreased plasma oncotic pressure, increased capillary permeability, and increased interstitial oncotic pressure or lymphatic obstruction. The major causes of each of these forces are reviewed below.

Edema may be benign or may indicate a life-threatening disease. As such, the etiology of edema should always be determined. Edema may be confined to one extremity or may be generalized and massive.

Causes of Peripheral Edema

Increased capillary hydraulic pressure

- Acute pulmonary edema
- Cirrhosis
- Compartment syndrome
- Compression of inferior vena cava or iliac veins
- Constrictive pericarditis
- Deep venous thrombosis
- Drugs (see below)
- Heart failure (right ventricular failure)
- Hepatic venous obstruction
- Pregnancy
- Premenstrual edema
- Primary renal sodium retention
- Refeeding edema
- Renal disease and nephritic syndrome
- Restrictive cardiomyopathy
- Tricuspid valvular disease
- Venous obstruction in an extremity

Decreased plasma oncotic pressure

- Cirrhosis
- Malabsorption
- Malnutrition
- Nephrotic syndrome
- Preeclampsia

Increased capillary permeability

- Adult respiratory distress syndrome
- Allergic reactions
- Burns
- Inflammation or local infections
- Interleukin-2 therapy
- Malignant ascites
- Trauma

Lymphatic obstruction or increased interstitial oncotic pressure

- Filariasis
- Hypothyroidism
- Malignant ascites
- Nodal enlargement from malignancy
- Post-radiation
- Postsurgical

Other

- Idiopathic
- Medications
- Myxedema

Medications Associated with Peripheral Edema

Antidepressants

Beta blockers

Calcium channel blockers (particularly dihydropyridines)

Centrally acting antihypertensives (clonidine, methyldopa)

Corticosteroids

COX-2 inhibitors

Docetaxel

Estrogens

Fludrocortisone

Guanethidine

Monoamine oxidase inhibitors

NSAIDs

Phenylbutazone

Pramipexole

Progesterones

Reserpine

Testosterone

Thiazolidinediones (pioglitazone, rosiglitazone)

Vasodilators (diazoxide, hydralazine, minoxidil)

Suggested Work-Up

Electrolytes, BUN, creatinine, and urinalysis	To evaluate renal function
Liver function tests	To evaluate for hepatic disease
Albumin level	To assess nutritional status and detect hepatic synthetic dysfunction
Thyroid-stimulating hormone	To evaluate for hypothyroidism
Electrocardiogram and chest X-ray	To evaluate for cardiopulmonary disease

Additional Work-Up

The following studies may be indicated when preliminary findings warrant them.

B-type natriuretic peptide	To evaluate for heart failure
Serum and protein electrophoresis	To evaluate for multiple myeloma
Complete thyroid function studies	To further evaluate thyroid abnormalities
24-hour urine collection or spot urine protein to creatinine ratio	To quantify the amount of proteinuria if proteinuria is found on the urinalysis
Imaging studies such as CT or echocardiography	If warranted based upon clinical findings
Invasive studies such as cardiac catheterization or biopsy	If warranted based upon clinical findings

Further reading

Cho S, Atwood JE. Peripheral edema. American Journal of Medicine 2002;113: 580–586.

Davison JM. Edema in pregnancy. Kidney International 1997;51(suppl): S90–S96.

Halperin AK, Cubeddu LX. The role of calcium channel blockers in the treatment of hypertension. American Heart Journal 1986;111: 363–382.

Markham RV Jr, Gilmore A, Pettinger WA, et al. Central and regional hemodynamic effects and neurohumoral consequences of minoxidil in severe congestive heart failure and comparison to hydralazine and nitroprusside. American Journal of Cardiology 1983; 52: 774–781.

O'Brien JG, Chennubhotla RV. Treatment of edema. American Family Physician 2005;71: 2111–2117.

Rose BD. Renal pathophysiology: the essentials. Baltimore: Williams & Wilkins; 1994.

Rose BD. Pathophysiology and etiology of edema. In: Rose BD, ed. UpToDate. Wellesley: UpToDate; 2004.

Thomas ML, Lloyd SJ. Pulmonary edema associated with rosiglitazone and troglitazone. Annals of Pharmacotherapy 2001;35: 123–124.

Valentin JP, Ribstein J, Halimi JM, et al. Effect of different calcium antagonists on transcapillary fluid shift. American Journal of Hypertension 1990;3: 491–495.

54 PERIPHERAL NEUROPATHY

General Discussion

Peripheral neuropathy represents one of the most common neurologic disorders encountered by primary care physicians. Peripheral neuropathy may be the result of hereditary, toxic, infectious, inflammatory, metabolic, ischemic, or paraneoplastic causes. Diabetes and alcoholism are the most common etiologies of peripheral neuropathy in adults living in developed countries. Despite extensive evaluation, an etiology is not found in 13–22% of cases.

Most patients can be diagnosed, classified, and managed based on the history and physical examination. Classifying the patient's neuropathy clinically based upon time course (acute, subacute, chronic, or lifelong), functional modalities affected (motor or sensory) and the distribution (distal, proximal, or patchy) can assist in diagnosis. Other important information includes medication use, past medical history, age of onset, and family history.

Medications Associated with Neuropathy

Alfa interferon

Amiodarone

Amitriptyline

Chloramphenicol

Chloroquine

Cimetidine

Cisplatin

Colchicine

Dapsone

Didanosine

Dideoxycytidine

Dideoxyinosine

Disulfiram

Docetaxel

Ethambutol

Gold

Hydralazine

Isoniazid

Lithium

Metronidazole

Nitrofurantoin

Nitrous oxide

Paclitaxel

Phenytoin

Pyridoxine (vitamin B$_6$)

Simvastatin

Suramin

Thalidomide

Vincristine

Causes of Peripheral Neuropathy

Acute pandysautonomia

Alcoholism

Amyloidosis

Carcinomatous axonal sensorimotor polyneuropathy

Chronic gluten enteropathy

Chronic inflammatory demyelinating polyradiculopathy

Crohn's disease

Churg–Strauss vasculitis

Compressive neuropathies

Critical illness polyneuropathy

Cryoglobulinemia

Diabetes mellitus

Diphtheria

Entrapment

- Acromegaly
- Amyloidosis
- Myxedema
- Rheumatoid arthritis

Folate deficiency

Friedreich's ataxia

Gastric restriction surgery for obesity

Gouty neuropathy

Guillain–Barré syndrome

Hereditary motor sensory neuropathy

HIV/AIDS

Hypophosphatemia

Hypothyroidism

Idiopathic sensory neuronopathy

Ischemic lesions

Leprosy

Lyme disease

Lymphoma

Lymphomatous axonal sensorimotor polyneuropathy

Metal neuropathy

- Acute arsenic polyneuropathy
- Chronic arsenic intoxication
- Lead neuropathy
- Mercury
- Gold
- Thallium

Monoclonal gammopathy of undetermined significance

Neoplastic infiltration or compression

Osteosclerotic myeloma

Paraneoplastic neuropathy

Paraproteinemias

Polyarteritis nodosa

Porphyria

Postgastrectomy syndrome

Primary biliary cirrhosis

Rheumatoid arthritis

Sarcoidosis

Sjögren's syndrome

Styrene-induced peripheral neuropathy

Systemic lupus erythematosus

Thiamine deficiency

Toxic neuropathy

- Acrylamide
- Carbon disulfide
- Carbon monoxide
- Dichlorophenoxyacetic acid
- Ethylene oxide
- Glue sniffing
- Hexacarbons
- Organophosphorus esters

Trauma

Vasculitis

Vitamin B$_{12}$ deficiency

Vitamin E deficiency

Waldenstrom's macroglobulinemia

Whipple's disease

Suggested Work-Up

EMG and nerve conduction studies (NCS)	Used to confirm the presence of a neuropathy and provide information regarding the type of fibers involved, the pathophysiology, and a symmetric versus asymmetric or multifocal pattern
Fasting serum glucose and glycosylated hemoglobin	To evaluate for diabetes mellitus
AST and ALT	To evaluate for occult alcoholism
Blood urea nitrogen and creatinine	To evaluate renal function
CBC	To evaluate for evidence of infection
ESR, ANA, rheumatoid factor	To evaluate for inflammatory and rheumatologic disorders
Urinalysis	To evaluate renal function
Vitamin B$_{12}$ level	To evaluate for B$_{12}$ deficiency
TSH level	To evaluate for thyroid abnormalities
Serum and urine protein electrophoresis	To evaluate for paraproteinemic neuropathies
Neurologic consultation should be obtained early for any acute progressive neuropathy	
For the patient with acute progressive neuropathy, EMG/NCS, electrocardiogram, lumbar puncture, chest radiograph, and pulmonary function tests are often performed	

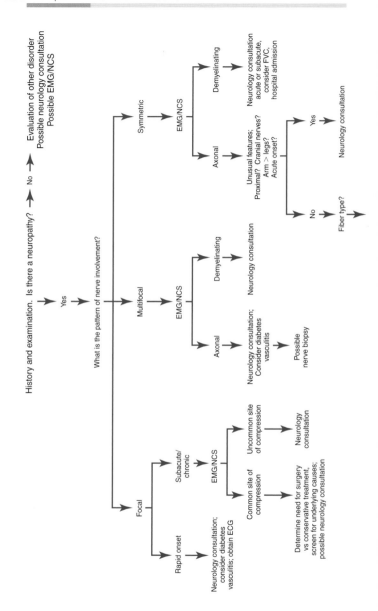

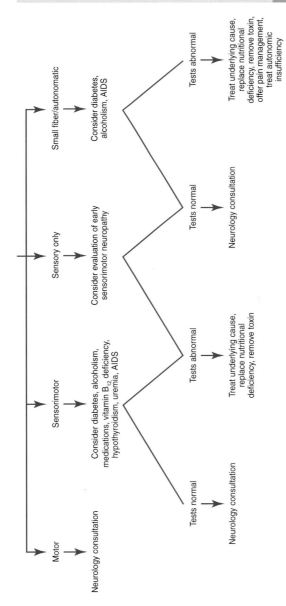

Figure 54-1. Algorithm for evaluation of a patient with a peripheral neuropathy. (ECG=electrocardiogram; EMG/NCS=electron microscopy/nerve conduction studies; AIDS=acquired immunodeficiency syndrome; FVC=forced vital capacity.)

Additional Selected Work-Up

Cerebrospinal fluid analysis	Useful in the evaluation of myelinopathies and polyradiculopathies
Lyme PCR	When Lyme disease is suspected
Cytomegalovirus branched chain DNA	For polyradiculopathy or mononeuritis multiplex in AIDS
Cytology	When lymphoma is suspected
Nerve biopsy	Used in specific cases to diagnose vasculitis, leprosy, amyloid neuropathy, leukodystrophies, and sarcoidosis.

Further reading

Chalk CH. Acquired neuromuscular diseases; acquired peripheral neuropathy. Neurologic Clinics 1997;15: 501–528.

Dyck PJ, Oviatt KF, Lambert EH. Intensive evaluation of referred unclassified neuropathies yields improved diagnosis. Annals of Neurology 1981;10: 222–226.

Griffin JW, Hsieh ST, McArthur JC, et al. Diagnostic testing in neurology: laboratory testing in peripheral nerve disease. Neurologic Clinics 1996;14: 119–133.

McLeod JG, Tuck RR, Pollard JD, et al. Chronic polyneuropathy of undetermined cause. Journal of Neurology, Neurosurgery, and Psychiatry 1984;47: 530–535.

Poncelet, AN. An algorithm for the evaluation of peripheral neuropathy. American Family Physician 1998;57: 755–764.

Sabin TD, Swift TR, Jacobson RR. Leprosy. In: Dyck PJ, Thomas PK, eds. Peripheral neuropathy. Philadelphia: Saunders; 1993:1354–1379.

General Discussion

Potential mechanisms of pleural fluid accumulation include increased interstitial fluid in the lungs secondary to increased pulmonary capillary pressure or permeability, decreased intrapleural pressure, decreased plasma oncotic pressure, increased pleural membrane permeability, obstructed lymphatic flow, diaphragmatic defects, and thoracic duct rupture. The most common causes in adults are heart failure, malignancy, pneumonia, tuberculosis, and pulmonary embolism. Heart failure is the most common cause of bilateral pleural effusion. However, if cardiomegaly is not seen with bilateral pleural effusion, other causes such as malignancy should be pursued.

The first step in identifying the underlying cause of a pleural effusion is determining whether the effusion is exudative or transudative. Thoracentesis should be performed in all patients with more than a minimal pleural effusion unless heart failure is the clear diagnosis. If heart failure is present, thoracentesis may be indicated if atypical circumstances are present such as fevers, pleuritic chest pain, unilateral effusion, effusions of markedly disparate size, cardiomegaly is not present, or if the effusion does not respond to treatment for heart failure.

Exudative effusions can be differentiated from transudative effusions using Light's criteria. Light's criteria are nearly 100% sensitive at identifying exudates. An effusion is an exudate if one or more of the following criteria are present:

- Pleural fluid lactate dehydrogenase (LDH) >two-thirds the upper limit of normal for serum LDH, or
- Pleural fluid-to-serum LDH ratio > 0.6, or
- Pleural fluid-to-serum protein ratio > 0.5

A patient with heart failure who has received diuretics may fulfill criteria for an exudative effusion. In this case, if the difference between protein levels in the serum and the pleural fluid is greater than 3.1 g/dL, the patient actually has a transudative effusion.

Additional tests used to identify an exudative pleural effusion include the following:

- Pleural fluid-serum albumin gradient >1.2 g/dL
- Pleural fluid-to-serum cholesterol ratio > 0.3

Any drug should be considered as a potential cause for an undiagnosed exudative effusion before pursuing an extensive diagnostic evaluation. The presentation of drug-induced pleural disease may vary from an asymptomatic pleural effusion to acute pleuritis to symptomatic pleural thickening. Pleural disease due to medications may occur as a result of hypersensitivity or allergic reaction, direct toxic effect, increased oxygen free radical production, suppression of antioxidant defenses, or chemical-induced inflammation. Pleural fluid eosinophilia, defined as > 10% of nucleated cells, may provide evidence for the presence of drug-induced pleural disease. However, the presence or absence of eosinophilia in the pleural fluid is a nonspecific finding. Other causes of pleural fluid eosinophilia include pneumothorax, fungal disease, parasitic infection, hemothorax, Hodgkin's lymphoma, benign asbestos pleural effusion, and pulmonary emboli with pulmonary infarction.

Medications Associated with Pleural Effusion

Absolute alcohol

Acyclovir

Amiodarone

Bleomycin

Bromocriptine

Clozapine

Cyclophosphamide

Dantrolene

Docetaxel

D-penicillamine

Gliclazide

Granulocyte colony-stimulating factor (G-CSF)

Interleukin-2

Intravenous immunoglobulin

Isotretinoin

Itraconazole

L-tryptophan

Mesalamine

Methotrexate

Methysergide

Minoxidil

Mitomycin

Nitrofurantoin

Oxyprenolol

Practolol

Procarbazine

Propylthiouracil

Simvastatin

Sodium morrhuate

Troglitazone

Valproic acid

Causes of Pleural Effusion

Atelectasis

Benign asbestos pleural effusion

Chylothorax

Cirrhosis

Dressler's syndrome

Duropleural fistula

Empyema

Esophageal perforation

Heart failure

Hemothorax

Hepatic hydrothorax

Hypoalbuminemia

Kaposi sarcoma

Lupus pleuritis

Lymphoma

Medications

Meigs' syndrome

Mesothelioma

Ovarian cancer

Ovarian hyperstimulation syndrome

Pancreatic effusion

Pericarditis

Pleural infection

Pleural malignancy

Pneumonia

Postoperative pleural effusion (especially after coronary artery bypass graft surgery)

Postpartum pleural effusion

Pseudochylothorax

Pulmonary embolism

Rheumatoid pleuritis

Subphrenic abscess

Trapped lung

Tuberculosis

Uremia

Viral disease

Yellow nail syndrome

Key Historical Features

✓ Cough

✓ Dyspnea

✓ Pleuritic chest pain

✓ Fevers

✓ Past medical history

✓ Past surgical history

✓ Medications

✓ Family history

✓ Social history

Key Physical Findings

✓ Vital signs

✓ General appearance

✓ Cardiac examination for evidence of heart failure

✓ Pulmonary examination for dullness to percussion, decreased or absent tactile fremitus, or decreased breath sounds

✓ Abdominal examination for hepatosplenomegaly, ascites, or masses

✓ Pelvic examination if ovarian malignancy is a potential diagnosis

Suggested Work-Up

Chest X-ray	To confirm the presence of a pleural effusion
Thoracentesis with pleural fluid sent for cell count and differential, glucose, cytology, LDH, and protein	Routine tests on pleural fluid
Pleural fluid pH and bacterial cultures	If infection is a possible diagnosis
Serum LDH and protein	Used to derive pleural fluid-to-serum ratios

| Polymerase chain reaction for *Mycobacterium tuberculosis* | If tuberculosis is suspected |

Additional Work-Up

Ultrasound or CT	If doubt exists about the pleural effusion, to detect small effusions, and to differentiate pleural fluid from pleural thickening. CT may be used in a patient suspected of having pulmonary embolism
Pleural fluid amylase	If esophageal rupture or pancreatic disease is suspected
Pleural fluid adenosine deaminase (ADA)	If tuberculosis is suspected
Pleural fluid cholesterol	If chylothorax or pseudochylothorax is suspected. May also be used to differentiate exudate from transudate
Hematocrit fluid:blood ratio	If pleural fluid is bloody to evaluate for hemothorax
Bronchoscopy	Useful when an endobronchial malignancy is suspected
Pleural biopsy	Useful when an exudative effusion remains undiagnosed or when tuberculosis or malignancy is suspected
Thoracoscopy	Useful in cytology-negative pleural effusion when pleural malignancy is suspected

Further reading

Burgess L, Maritz FJ, Taljaard JF. Comparative analysis of the biochemical parameters used to distinguish between pleural transudates and exudates. Chest 1995;107: 1604.

Heffner JE. Evaluating diagnostic tests in the pleural space: differentiating transudates from exudates as a model. Clinics in Chest Medicine 1998;19: 277–293.

Huggins JT, Sahn SA. Drug-induced pleural disease. Clinics in Chest Medicine 2004;25: 141–153.

Morelock SY, Sahn SA. Drugs and the pleura. Chest 1999;116: 212–221.

Porcel JM, Light RW. Diagnostic approach to pleural effusion in adults. American Family Physician 2006;73: 1211–1220.

General Discussion

The effective preoperative evaluation seeks to perform several tasks which include (1) decreasing surgical morbidity; (2) minimizing expensive delays and cancellations on the day of surgery; (3) evaluating and optimizing patient health status; (4) facilitating the planning of anesthesia and perioperative care; and (5) reducing patient anxiety through education. The complete consultation should include recommendations for evaluation and treatment, including prophylactic therapies to minimize the perioperative risk.

Surgical complications occur frequently and generally include cardiac, respiratory, and infectious complications. The overall risk for surgical complications depends on individual factors and the type of surgical procedure being considered. Diseases associated with an increased risk for surgical complications include respiratory disease, cardiac disease, diabetes mellitus, and malnutrition. Cardiac complications are the most common cause of morbidity and mortality in the surgical patient.

Ideally, the patient should be evaluated several weeks before the planned surgical procedure. Emergency surgery requires expedited preoperative cardiac assessment and management. Patients undergoing elective or semielective procedures can proceed with preoperative cardiac testing if indicated.

The patient's medical history usually is the most important component of the preoperative evaluation. The value of routine medical testing before elective surgery is unclear because most abnormalities in laboratory values can be predicted from the patient's history and findings on the physical examination. Current recommendations call for fewer routine tests and instead recommend selective ordering of laboratory tests based on the specific indication in a given patient.

Aspirin and NSAIDs should be discontinued 1 week before surgery to minimize the risk of excessive bleeding. If the patient smokes, the patient should quit smoking at least 8 weeks before surgery to minimize the surgical risks associated with smoking.

Recommendations do not call for preoperative cardiac testing in all patients. The need for cardiac evaluation is determined by the clinical risk factors identified from the patient's history, physical examination, functional status, EKG, and the risks inherent to the procedure being considered. Figure 56.1 provides the guidelines of the American College of Cardiology and the American Heart Association.

The role for preoperative pulmonary function testing remains controversial. The American College of Physicians recommends spirometry in patients with a history of dyspnea and tobacco use who are undergoing upper abdominal or coronary artery bypass surgery. For any patient with cough or dyspnea, a work-up should be performed to evaluate for the underlying etiology. Asthma should be under control before surgery if possible. Any pulmonary infection should be treated preoperatively.

All patients with coronary artery disease (CAD) and possibly those with risk factors for CAD should receive perioperative beta blockers unless a strong contraindication exists.

Key Historical Features

✓ Surgical procedure being considered

✓ Past medical history, especially heart and lung disease

- Coronary artery disease
- Previous cardiovascular procedural interventions or testing
- Symptoms suggestive of angina or congestive heart failure

✓ Past surgical history

✓ Anesthetic history

✓ Medications, including over-the-counter medications and herbal supplements

✓ Recent use of anticoagulants, aspirin, or NSAIDs

✓ Allergies to medications

✓ Smoking history

✓ Alcohol or drug use

✓ Complete review of systems, especially cough, dyspnea, and chest pain

✓ Functional status

✓ Self-reported exercise tolerance

✓ Risk factors for malnutrition such as social isolation, limited financial resources, poor dentition, and weight loss

Key Physical Findings

✓ Vital signs

✓ Cardiac examination for evidence of heart murmurs, signs of congestive heart failure, or cardiovascular disease

✓ Pulmonary examination for evidence of pulmonary disease

✓ Evidence of malnutrition

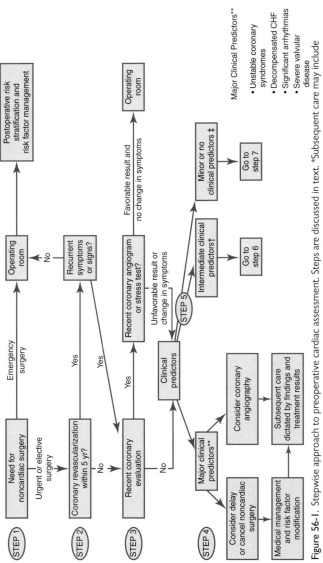

Figure 56-1. Stepwise approach to preoperative cardiac assessment. Steps are discussed in text. *Subsequent care may include cancellation or delay of surgery, coronary revascularization followed by noncardiac surgery, or intensified care. CHF indicates congestive heart failure; ECG, electrocardiogram; MET, metabolic equivalent; MI, myocardial infarction.

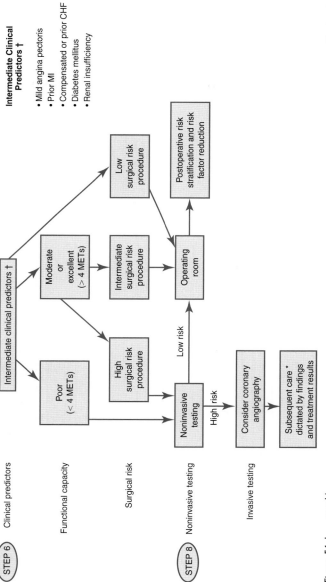

Continued

Figure 56-1. —cont'd

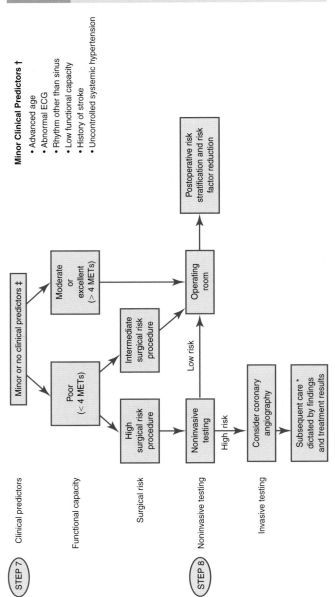

Figure 56-1. —cont'd

Suggested Work-Up

Hemoglobin and pregnancy test for women of childbearing age   For patients under 40 years of age

Hemoglobin, blood glucose, pregnancy test for women of childbearing age, and EKG   For patients over 40–45 years of age

Additional Work-Up

Albumin and total lymphocyte   For patients with evidence of malnutrition. Serum count albumin <3.2 mg/dL or a total lymphocyte count <3000/μL may signify malnutrition

EKG, chest X-ray, hemoglobin, electrolytes, BUN, creatinine, glucose   For patients with evidence of cardiovascular disease or patients with history of diabetes

Echocardiogram   For patients in whom decreased left ventricular function is suspected on the basis of the history, examination, or radiographic evidence of cardiac enlargement

Cardiology consultation   For patients with myocardial infarction in the last 6 weeks, unstable angina, decompensated CHF, significant arrhythmias, or severe vascular disease

Stress test if high-risk procedure or patient has low functional capacity   For patients with history of myocardial infarction more than 6 weeks ago, mild stable angina, compensated CHF, or diabetes mellitus

Stress test if high-risk procedure and patient has low functional capacity   For patients with cardiac rhythm other than normal sinus rhythm, abnormal EKG, history of CVA, advanced age, or low functional capacity

Chest radiographs, hemoglobin, glucose, EKG   For patients with pulmonary disease

Pulmonary function testing   Should be considered in patients with asthma, COPD

Further reading

American Heart Association. Guidelines for perioperative cardiovascular evaluation for noncardiac surgery: report of the American College of Cardiology/American Heart Association Task Force on Practice Guidelines (Committee on Perioperative Cardiovascular Evaluation for Noncardiac Surgery). Circulation 1996;93: 1278–1317.

American Heart Association. ACC/AHA Guideline Update for Perioperative Cardiovascular Evaluation for Noncardiac Surgery-Executive Summary. A Report of the American College of Cardiology/American Heart Association Task Force on Practice Guidelines (Committee to Update the 1996 Guidelines on Perioperative Cardiovascular Evaluation for Noncardiac Surgery). Circulation 2002;105: 1257–1267.

Fischer SP. Cost-effective preoperative evaluation and testing. Chest 1999;115: 96–100.

King MS. Preoperative evaluation. American Family Physician 2000;62: 387–396.

Michota FA, Frost SD. Perioperative management of the hospitalized patient. Medical Clinics of North America 2002;86: 731–748.

General Discussion

Proteinuria is a frequent finding on dipstick testing of urine specimens, yet fewer than 2% of these represent serious and treatable urinary tract disorders. Proteinuria is defined as urinary protein excretion of greater than 150 mg per day and can be classified pathophysiologically as glomerular, tubular, or overflow.

Causes of false-positive results include prolonged immersion of the dipstick, highly concentrated urine, alkaline urine, gross hematuria, the use of penicillin, sulfonamides, or tolbutamide, or the presence of semen, vaginal secretions, or pus.

If proteinuria is found on a dipstick urinalysis, the urinary sediment should be examined microscopically. Findings on the microscopic urinalysis are outlined below. If the dipstick urinalysis shows trace to 2+ protein and the results of the microscopic urinalysis are inconclusive, the dipstick test should be repeated on a morning specimen at least twice during the next month. If a subsequent dipstick test is negative, the patient has transient proteinuria, which is associated with high fevers, hard exercise, and CHF. Transient proteinuria does not require follow-up.

If the dipstick urinalysis shows persistent proteinuria or if proteinuria of 3+ or 4+ is found, the evaluation should proceed to a quantitative evaluation of a specimen. Quantitative measurement of protein excretion can be performed with a urine protein:creatinine ratio in a random urine specimen or a 24-hour urine specimen.

Persons younger than 30 years who excrete less than 2 grams of protein per day and who have a normal creatinine clearance should be tested for orthostatic (postural) proteinuria. This is a benign condition associated with prolonged standing that is confirmed with a negative urinalysis result after 8 hours of recumbency.

The diagnosis of isolated proteinuria can be made in a patient who has proteinuria less than 2 grams per day with normal renal function, no evidence of systemic disease affecting renal function, a normal urine sediment, and normal blood pressure. These patients should be observed with blood pressure measurement, urinalysis, and creatinine clearance every 6 months.

An adult with proteinuria greater than 2 grams per 24 hours or with proteinuria and decreased creatinine clearance requires aggressive work-up in consultation with a nephrologist. If the creatinine clearance is normal and the patient has a medical diagnosis such as CHF or diabetes mellitus, the underlying disease can be treated with close monitoring of the proteinuria and renal function. A consultation with a nephrologist should be considered if the renal function or amount of proteinuria changes.

Causes of Proteinuria

Overflow proteinuria

- Amyloidosis
- Hemoglobinuria
- Multiple myeloma
- Myoglobinuria

Primary glomerular causes

- Focal segmental glomerulonephritis
- Idiopathic membranous glomerulonephritis
- IgA nephropathy
- IgM nephropathy
- Membranoproliferative glomerulonephritis
- Membranous nephropathy
- Minimal change disease

Secondary glomerular causes

- Alport's syndrome
- Amyloidosis
- Diabetes mellitus
- Drugs
  - ACE inhibitors
  - Gold
  - Heavy metals
  - Heroin
  - Lithium
  - NSAIDs
  - Penicillamine
- Fabry's disease
- Infection
  - Endocarditis
  - Hepatitis B
  - Hepatitis C
  - HIV
  - Leprosy
  - Malaria
  - Parasitic diseases
  - Post streptococcal infection
  - Shunt nephritis
  - Syphilis

- Malignancy (lymphoma, solid tumors)
- Preeclampsia
- Sarcoidosis
- Sickle cell disease
- Systemic lupus erythematosus and other collagen vascular diseases

Transient proteinuria

- Congestive heart failure
- Dehydration
- Emotional distress
- Exercise
- Fever
- Orthostatic (postural proteinuria)
- Seizures

Tubular causes

- Aminoaciduria
- Drugs
  - Antibiotics
  - NSAIDs
- Fanconi syndrome
- Heavy metal ingestion
- Hypertensive nephrosclerosis
- Interstitial nephritis
- Sickle cell disease
- Uric acid nephropathy

Key Historical Features

✓ Recent illness or fever

✓ Facial or extremity swelling

✓ Medical history, especially those listed above that are causes of proteinuria

✓ Medications

✓ Exercise habits

✓ Risk factors for sexually transmitted diseases

✓ Heavy metal exposure

Key Physical Findings

✓ Vital signs, especially evidence of hypertension

✓ Signs of systemic disease

✓ Funduscopic examination

✓ Cardiovascular examination

✓ Pulmonary examination

✓ Abdominal examination, including bruits

✓ Edema (periorbital or peripheral)

✓ Rash

Suggested Work-Up

Microscopic examination of urine sediment	Fatty casts or oval fat bodies suggest nephrotic syndrome
	Leukocytes, or leukocyte casts with bacteria suggest urinary tract infection
	Leukocytes or leukocyte casts without bacteria suggest renal interstitial disease
	Normal red cells suggest a lower urinary tract lesion
	Dysmorphic red cells suggest an upper urinary tract lesion
	Red cell casts suggest glomerular disease
	Waxy, granular, or cellular casts suggest advanced chronic renal disease
	Eosinophils suggest drug-induced acute interstitial nephritis
	Hyaline casts are not suggestive of renal disease but are present with dehydration and diuretic therapy
24-hour urine specimen or spot measurement of protein: creatinine ratio	To quantitate protein excretion

Antinuclear antibody	Elevated in systemic lupus erythematosus
Antistreptolysin O titer	Elevated levels indicated post-streptococcal glomerulonephritis
Complement C3 and C4	Levels decreased in glomerulonephritides
Erythrocyte sedimentation rate	Elevation may indicate inflammatory or infectious causes
Fasting serum glucose	To evaluate for diabetes mellitus
CBC	Anemia may indicate chronic renal failure
HIV, VDRL, hepatitis B and hepatitis C serologies	HIV, syphilis, hepatitis B, and hepatitis C are associated with glomerular proteinuria
Serum albumin and lipids	Albumin is decreased and cholesterol level is increased in nephrotic syndrome
Serum electrolytes, calcium and phosphorus	Provide screening for any abnormalities following renal disease
Serum and urine protein electrophoresis	To rule out multiple myeloma
Serum urate	Elevated urate can cause tubulointerstitial disease
Renal ultrasound	To evaluate for structural renal disease
Chest x-ray	To examine for systemic disease such as sarcoidosis

Additional Work-Up

Renal biopsy	Usually recommended for nephrotic range proteinuria (>3.5 g in 24 hours)

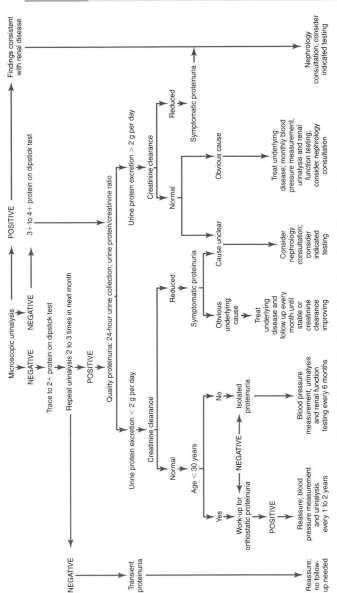

Figure 57-1. Algorithm for evaluating the patient with proteinuria.

Further reading

Ahmed Z, Lee J. Asymptomatic urinary abnormalities: hematuria and proteinuria. Medical Clinics of North America 1997;81: 641–652.

Carroll MF, Temte JL. Proteinuria in adults: a diagnostic approach. American Family Physician 2000;62: 1333–1340.

Glassrock RJ. Proteinuria. In: Massry SJ, Glassrock RJ, eds. Textbook of nephrology, 3rd ed. Baltimore: Williams & Wilkins; 1995:602.

Simerville JA, Maxted WC, Pahira JJ. Urinalysis: a comprehensive review. American Family Physician 2005;71: 1153–1162.

Woolhandler S, Pels RJ, Bor DH, et al. Dipstick urinalysis screening of asymptomatic adults for urinary tract disorders: hematuria and proteinuria. Journal of the American Medical Association 1989;262: 1214–1219.

58 PRURITUS

General Discussion

The sensation of itching, or pruritus, is the most common symptom of dermatologic conditions, but may also be associated with systemic disease, even in the absence of primary cutaneous findings. Histamine is the main mediator of itching, but other mediators may be involved, including serotonin, neuropeptides, and prostaglandins.

Pruritus is frequently encountered as a symptom of common dermatologic conditions such as atopic dermatitis, contact dermatitis, psoriasis, and urticaria. Additional dermatologic causes of itching are outlined below. When primary skin findings are absent, the approach shifts to attempting to detect an underlying systemic disorder. In patients with pruritus, the prevalence of underlying systemic disease ranges from 10% to 50%. If no specific dermatologic disorder is identified after a thorough history and physical examination, laboratory and radiologic tests should be ordered to try to identify the presence of systemic disease.

Medications That Cause Cholestasis or Cholestatic Hepatitis

Allopurinol

Ampicillin

Anabolic steroids

Antibiotics

- Amoxicillin/clavulanic acid
- Azithromycin
- Clarithromycin
- Dapsone
- Erythromycin
- Flucloxacillin
- Nitrofurantoin
- Trimethoprim/sulfamethoxazol

Arsenic

Azathioprine

Barbiturates

Benzodiazepines

Captopril

Carbamazepine

Chlorpromazine

Chlorpropamide

Cimetidine

Clindamycin

Co-trimoxazole

Cyclohexylpropionate

Cyclosporin A

Cyproheptadine

Cytosine-arabinoside

Danazol

Erythromycin

Fosinopril

Gold

Haloperidol

Infliximab

Loracarbef

Mesalamine

Methimazole

Nifedipine

NSAIDs

- Diclofenac
- Ibuprofen
- Nimesulide
- Sulindac

Phenytoin

Pizotyline

Prochlorperazine

Propoxyphene

Risperidone

Sex steroids

Tamoxifen

Terbinafine

Terfenadine

Tetracyclines

Thiabendazole

Tricyclic antidepressants

Troglitazone

Conditions Associated with Pruritus

Acquired immunodeficiency syndrome

Advanced age

Anorexia nervosa

Cutaneous mastocytosis

Dermatologic conditions

- Atopic dermatitis
- Bullous pemphigoid
- Contact dermatitis
- Dermatitis herpetiformis
- Miliaria
- Parasitic infestations
- Pruritus ani/scroti/vulvi
- Psoriasis
- Urticaria
- Xerosis

Endocrine disorders

- Carcinoid syndrome
- Diabetes mellitus
- Hyperthyroidism
- Hypothyroidism
- Multiple endocrine neoplasia type 2

Hematopoietic diseases

- Hodgkin's disease
- Iron-deficiency anemia
- Leukemia
- Lymphoma
- Mastocytosis
- Mycosis fungoides
- Plasma cell dyscrasias
- Polycythemia vera

Linear IgA dermatosis

Liver and biliary disease

- Drug-induced cholestasis
- Extrahepatic biliary obstruction
- Infectious hepatitis
- Primary biliary cirrhosis
- Pruritus gravidarum
- Sclerosing cholangitis

Malignancy

Medications

Neurologic disorders
- Cerebral abscess
- Cerebral tumor
- Multiple sclerosis
- Stroke

Psychiatric illness

Renal disease
- Chronic renal failure

Key Historical Features

✓ Duration and quality of the itching

✓ Distribution of itching

✓ Exacerbating and ameliorating factors

✓ Past medical history

✓ Medications

✓ Illicit drug use

✓ Personal or family history of atopy or skin disease

✓ Occupation and hobbies

✓ Environmental exposures

✓ Animal exposure

✓ Travel history

✓ Sexual history

✓ Bathing habits

✓ Thorough review of systems

Key Physical Findings

✓ Thorough skin examination for rash, excoriations, dyspigmentation, or lichenification

✓ Palpation of lymph nodes for lymphadenopathy

✓ Palpation of liver and spleen for organomegaly

✓ Inspection of fingers, axillae, and genitals to evaluate for scabies

Suggested Work-Up

CBC with differential	To evaluate for hematopoietic disorders
AST, ALT, bilirubin, GGT, albumin	To evaluate for hepatobiliary disease
BUN and creatinine	To evaluate for renal disease
TSH	To evaluate for hypo- or hyperthyroidism
Plasma glucose	To evaluate for diabetes mellitus
Urinalysis	To evaluate for renal disease
Chest x-ray	To evaluate for pulmonary parasitic infestation
Stool for occult blood and parasites	To evaluate for intestinal parasitic infestation
HIV antibody	If risk factors for HIV infection are present

Additional Work-Up

Punch biopsy of the skin	May be considered if the cause of the itching cannot be determined from history, physical exam, and laboratory/radiologic evaluation

Further reading

Charlesworth EN, Beltrani VS. Pruritic dermatoses: overview of etiology and therapy. The American Journal of Medicine 2002;113(Suppl 9A): 255–335.

Etter L, Myers SA. Pruritis in systemic disease: mechanisms and management. Dermatology Clinics 2002;20: 459–472.

Kantor G, Lookingbill D. Generalized pruritis and systemic disease. Journal of the American Academy of Dermatology 1983;9: 375–382.

Krajnik M, Zylicz Z. Pruritis in advanced internal diseases: pathogenesis and treatment. The Netherlands Journal of Medicine 2001;58: 27–40.

Levy C, Lindor KD. Drug-induced cholestasis. Clinics in Liver Disease 2003;7: 7311–7330.

Yosipovitch G, David M. The diagnostic and therapeutic approach to idiopathic generalized pruritis. International Journal of Dermatology 1999;38: 881–887.

General Discussion

In the general population, urinary tract infection (UTI) is primarily an infection of sexually active women, with the prevalence of UTI in women outnumbering men by a ratio of 30:1. However, the prevalence of UTI increases in both sexes with advancing age, reducing the ratio to 2:1. Recurrent UTI is defined as three or more episodes of symptomatic bacteriuria within 1 year. A recurrent infection is one that occurs following documented, successful resolution of an antecedent infection.

In younger adults, recurrent infection occurs most often as a bladder infection in women, and is usually related to sexual intercourse. In older persons, recurrence is primarily a lower tract disease as a result of different risk or contributing factors, which may include incomplete bladder emptying or age-related diseases such as diabetes mellitus.

The decision to evaluate recurrent UTI radiologically, endoscopically, urodynamically, or otherwise should be based on the patient's clinical presentation, history, findings, response to antimicrobial therapy, and pattern of recurrent UTIs. A patient with a severe UTI warrants further evaluation. Severe UTI is defined as sepsis, fever, history of UTI lasting more than 7 days, gross hematuria, signs or symptoms of obstruction, or history of stones. Risk factors such as diabetes mellitus, immunosuppression, debilitating disease, or pregnancy also may warrant further evaluation.

If a patient has a history of recurrent UTI, urine culture should be used to document the infection, identify the pathogen, and determine the frequency of infection. Urine culture is also used to distinguish between unresolved and recurrent infection. If the same pathogen is documented repeatedly and at close intervals, an underlying abnormality should be suspected and an evaluation should be initiated. If the same pathogen is not found or UTIs do not occur in a close temporal relationship, the likelihood of the infections being associated with functional, metabolic, or anatomic abnormalities is low and the patient may be treated with low-dose antimicrobial prophylaxis. However, men with recurrent infections should be evaluated further because they usually are associated with an anatomic or functional urinary tract abnormality.

Conditions Associated with Recurrent UTI

Advancing age

Bacterial resistance

Chronic bacterial prostatitis

Diabetes mellitus

Genitourinary anatomic abnormalities (bladder polyp, urethral diverticula, fistula, medullary sponge kidney)

Genitourinary calculi

Immunosuppression

Incomplete bladder emptying (spinal cord injury, neurogenic bladder, advancing age)

Indwelling catheter

Medication noncompliance

Perinephric abscess

Pregnancy

Pyelonephritis

Poor hygiene

Renal abscess

Sexual intercourse

Urinary diversion procedure

Urologic instrumentation

Key Historical Features

✓ Age

✓ Previous response to therapy and culture results

✓ Presence of fever, nausea, or malaise

✓ Frequency of infection and temporal relationship to intercourse

✓ Contraceptive practices

✓ Dysuria

✓ Urinary frequency

✓ Urgency

✓ Hematuria

✓ Vaginal discharge

✓ Odor

✓ Dyspareunia

✓ Pruritis

✓ History of childhood infections

✓ Past medical history, especially urolithiasis, known urinary tract abnormality, immunosuppression, or diabetes mellitus

✓ Previous urologic surgery or instrumentation

Key Physical Findings

✓ Vital signs

✓ General examination to evaluate patient's overall health

✓ Abdominal examination

✓ Back examination to evaluate for costovertebral angle tenderness

✓ Genitourinary examination to evaluate for urethritis or vaginitis

✓ Gynecologic examination to rule out vaginal pathology

✓ Prostate examination

Suggested Work-Up

Urinalysis	To determine whether the urine is infected
Urine culture	To document infection, identify the pathogen, and determine the frequency of infection
BUN and creatinine	To evaluate renal function
Quantification of postvoid residual bladder volume	To evaluate bladder emptying
Renal ultrasound	To evaluate upper urinary tract architecture and establish the presence of hydronephrosis or abscess
or	
Intravenous pyelogram	To evaluate for filling defects or diagnose obstructive uropathy
or	
CT scan	To evaluate anatomic detail and to diagnose the presence of urinary stones

Additional Work-Up

Voiding cystogram	If an anatomical abnormality is suspected
Cystoscopy	If tumor or mass is suspected

Prostatic secretion wet mount or Gram stain	If chronic bacterial prostatitis is suspected in a male
Urology consult	For obstructive uropathy, calculi, abscess, or genitourinary abnormalities

Further reading

Engel JD, Schaeffer AJ. Evaluation of and antimicrobial therapy for recurrent urinary tract infections in women. Urologic Clinics of North America 1998;25:685–701.

McLaughlin SP, Carson CC. Urinary tract infections in women. Medical Clinics of North America 2004;88:417–429.

Pewitt EB, Schaeffer AJ. Urinary tract infection in urology, including acute and chronic prostatitis. Infectious Disease Clinics of North America 1997;11:623–646.

Yoshikawa TT, Nicolle LE, Norman DC. Management of complicated urinary tract infection in older patients. Journal of the American Geriatrics Society 1996;44:1235–1241.

General Discussion

Renal masses can be categorized into cysts, tumors, and inflammatory lesions. Autopsy results have shown that about 50% of persons older than 50 years have one or more renal cysts. Simple cysts usually are asymptomatic, but may cause flank pain, abdominal pain, hematuria, or a palpable mass. Malignant lesions may produce the same symptoms and may be associated with paraneoplastic syndromes. Inflammatory lesions are almost always associated with a history of fever, chills, or urinary tract infection.

Simple renal cysts must be distinguished from complex cysts and solid masses. The ultrasound criteria for the diagnosis of a simple renal cyst include the following:

(1) Spherical or ovoid shape.

(2) Absence of internal echoes.

(3) Presence of a thin, smooth wall that is separate from the surrounding parenchyma.

(4) Enhancement of the posterior wall, indicating ultrasound transmission through the water-filled cyst.

When these ultrasound criteria are met, the likelihood of malignancy is extremely small. Asymptomatic patients with incidental renal cysts that meet these criteria require no additional evaluation.

When visualization of the mass is inadequate on ultrasonography or when the ultrasound shows evidence of calcifications, septa, or multiple cysts that may obscure a potential malignancy, renal CT scanning with contrast should be performed.

Classification of Renal Masses

The Bosniak system is the most widely used categorization system for cystic renal masses. The system uses Houndsfield units (HU) to categorize lesions in order of increasing probability of malignancy.

Class I lesions are simple benign cysts. These lesions are round or oval in shape with no perceptible wall, have the same density as water, and exhibit no enhancement on radiographs taken after contrast medium is administered. No further evaluation is required. If the patient becomes symptomatic, as rarely occurs with large cysts, urologic consultation should be obtained.

Class II lesions are benign. These lesions include septated cysts, minimally calcified cysts, infected cysts, or cysts with higher density due to the presence of blood, protein, or colloid. These lesions should not enhance with

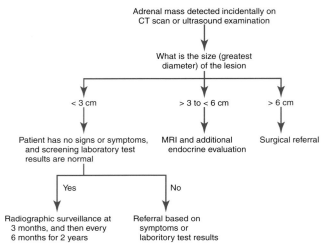

Figure 60-1. Management of incidental renal mass. (CT = computed tomographic scanning; MRI = magnetic resonance imaging.)

contrast medium and should be smaller than 3 cm in greatest diameter. Surveillance may be indicated because there is a small chance that these cysts may develop into renal cell carcinomas. Renal CT at 6- to 12-month intervals is suggested.

Class III lesions are more complicated cystic lesions with thick, irregular calcifications, multilocular form, thick irregular borders, thickened or enhancing septa, small nonenhancing nodules, or irregular calcifications. Urologic referral is indicated for these lesions. MRI may help to better characterize the lesions.

Class IV lesions are clearly malignant cystic masses. The lesions are heterogeneous with a shaggy appearance, thickened walls, or enhancing nodules resulting from necrosis and liquefaction of a solid tumor or a tumor growing in the wall. Surgical excision is indicated.

Further reading

Bosniak MA. The current radiologic approach to renal cysts. Radiology 1986:158: 1–10.
Curry NS, Bissada NK. Radiologic evaluation of small and indeterminant renal masses.
    The Urologic Clinics of North America 1997;24: 493–505.

Higgins JC, Fitzgerald JM. Evaluation of indidental renal and adrenal masses. American Family
    Physician 2001;63: 288–291.
Kissane JM. Congenital malformations. In: Jennette JC, Olson JL, Schwartz MM, Silva FG, eds.
    Heptinstall's pathology of the kidney, 5th ed. Philadelphia: Lippincott-Raven; 1998.
Wolf JS. Evaluation and management of solid and cystic renal masses. Journal of Urology
    1998;159: 1120–1133.

General Discussion

Rhinitis can be practically viewed as a heterogeneous group of nasal disorders characterized by symptoms such as rhinorrhea, nasal congestion, nasal itching, and sneezing. These classic symptoms of rhinitis overlap significantly in allergic rhinitis and other forms of rhinitis, as well as with various anatomic abnormalities of the upper airway. Rhinitis may be caused by allergic, nonallergic, hormonal, infectious, occupational, and other factors. Allergic rhinitis is the most common type of chronic rhinitis, though 30–50% of patients with rhinitis have nonallergic causes.

Allergic rhinitis can be categorized as seasonal, perennial, or occupational. Characteristics of allergic rhinitis include onset of symptoms early in life, a positive family history of allergic rhinitis, seasonal variability, itching in the nose, throat, or eyes, and the presence of identifiable suspected allergens. Physical examination often reveals moist and slightly blue nasal turbinates.

The diagnosis of nonallergic rhinitis is made after allergic or IgE-mediated causes have been eliminated. Characteristics that suggest nonallergic rhinitis include onset of symptoms after age 30, a negative family history of allergic rhinitis, perennial symptoms, the absence of nasal or throat itching, symptoms that are precipitated by irritants or weather changes, and the presence of viral or flu-like symptoms. Physical examination often reveals nasal mucosa that is dry, erythematous, or irritated.

Since 1998, three expert panels have published reviews of rhinitis. None of the three reports on rhinitis provides specific recommendations on when to perform allergy testing for patients with rhinitis. Empiric treatment is appropriate in patients with classic symptoms. In general, diagnostic tests may be appropriate if they will change outcomes, change treatment plans, if the symptoms are severe, if an unclear diagnosis is present, or if the patient is a potential candidate for allergen avoidance treatment or immunotherapy.

The most common diagnostic tests for allergic rhinitis are the percutaneous skin test and the allergen-specific immunoglobulin E (IgE) antibody test. Other diagnostic tools include nasal cytology and nasolaryngoscopy. Skin testing involves introducing allergen and control substances into the skin. The primary goal of skin testing is to detect the immediate allergic response caused by the release of mast cell or basophil IgE-specific mediators. Allergen-specific IgE antibody testing, also known as radioallergosorbent testing (RAST) is highly specific but not as sensitive as skin testing. RAST is useful for identifying common allergens such as pet dander, dust mites, pollen, and common molds but is less useful for identifying food, venom, and drug allergies. Generally speaking, skin testing or RAST testing should be used to confirm suspicions but should not be relied on to make a diagnosis.

Medications Associated with Rhinitis

ACE inhibitors

Anti-hypertensives

Aspirin

Beta blockers

Chlorpromazine

NSAIDs

Oral contraceptives

Causes of Rhinitis

Allergic rhinitis

- Occupational rhinitis
- Perennial rhinitis
- Seasonal rhinitis

Anatomic abnormalities

- Adenoidal hypertrophy
- Choanal atresia
- Foreign body in the nose
- Hypertrophic turbinates
- Nasal polyps
- Nasal tumors

Atrophic rhinitis

Cerebrospinal fluid leak

Cocaine abuse

Diabetes mellitus

Emotional rhinitis

Ethanol ingestion

Exercise-induced rhinitis

Gustatory

Hormonal

- Hypothyroidism
- Menstrual cycle
- Oral contraceptives
- Pregnancy

Infectious

Inflammatory or immunologic conditions

- Midline granuloma
- Nasal polyposis

- Sarcoidosis
- Septal deviation
- Sjögren's syndrome
- Systemic lupus erythematosus
- Wegener's granulomatosis

Medication-induced

Nonallergic rhinitis with eosinophilia syndrome (NARES)

Postural reflexes

Primary ciliary dyskinesia

Reflux-induced rhinitis (gastroesophageal reflux disease)

Relapsing polychondritis

Rhinitis medicamentosa

Vasomotor rhinitis

Key Historical Features

✓ Specific symptoms such as nasal congestion, rhinorrhea, sneezing, or pruritus

✓ Duration and chronicity

✓ Magnitude of reaction

✓ Eye itching and lacrimation

✓ Pattern of symptoms (intermittent, seasonal, perennial)

✓ Precipitating factors/triggers

✓ Response to medications

✓ Coexisting conditions

✓ Environmental history (home and occupational exposures)

✓ Past medical history, including trauma

✓ Medications

✓ Family history

Key Physical Findings

✓ Presence of fever

✓ Nasal examination for nasal discharge, swollen turbinates, bluish or pale mucosa, nasal polyps, septal deviation, and masses

✓ Ocular examination for conjunctivitis

✓ Evidence of infraorbital darkening or transverse nasal crease

✓ Ear examination for air–fluid levels

✓   Examination of the oropharynx for enlarged tonsils or pharyngeal postnasal discharge

✓   Neck examination for lymphadenopathy

✓   Pulmonary examination for evidence of asthma

✓   Skin examination for evidence of eczema

Suggested Work-Up

Empiric treatment is appropriate in patients with classic symptoms. In general, diagnostic tests may be appropriate if they will change outcomes, change treatment plans, if the symptoms are severe, if an unclear diagnosis is present, or if the patient is a potential candidate for allergen avoidance treatment or immunotherapy.

Skin testing	To identify specific allergens when avoidance measures or allergen immunotherapy are being considered
RAST	Highly specific but not as sensitive as skin testing. RAST is useful for identifying common allergens such as pet dander, dust mites, pollen, and common molds but is less useful for identifying food, venom, and drug allergies

Additional Work-Up

Nasal smear	Staining the nasal secretions for eosinophils with Hansel's stain can help suggest an allergic cause, but is not specific. Irritant and infectious rhinitis produce a neutrophil predominance

Further reading

Dykewicz MS. Allergic disorders. Journal of Allergy and Clinical Immunology 2003; 111: S520–S529.

Dykewicz MS, Fineman S, Skoner DP, et al. Diagnosis and management of rhinitis: complete guidelines of the Joint Task Force on Practice Parameters in Allergy, Asthma, and Immunology. American Academy of Allergy, Asthma, and Immunology. Annals of Allergy, Asthma & Immunology 1998;81(pt 2): 478–518.

Knight A. Anticholinergic therapy for allergic and nonallergic rhinitis and the common cold. Journal of Allergy and Clinical Immunology 1995;95: 1080–1083.

Quillen DM, Feller DB. Diagnosing rhinitis: allergic vs. nonallergic. American Family Physician 2006;73: 1583–1590.

Weldon D. Diagnosis and management of rhinitis. Primary Care: Clinics in Office Practice 1998;25: 831–848.

Wheeler PW, Wheeler SF. Vasomotor rhinitis. American Family Physician 2005;72: 1057–1062.

General Discussion

Seizures may be classified as localized (partial or focal) or generalized based upon clinical and electroencephalographic changes. A generalized seizure involves the cerebral hemispheres bilaterally and symmetrically at the time of onset. In contrast, a partial seizure originates in a specific region of the cerebral cortex. These seizures may be associated with signs or symptoms related to the cerebral region of origin, and they may occur with or without mental status changes or loss of consciousness.

Seizures have a bimodal frequency, declining in frequency from childhood until the age of 60 years, then increasing again. In adults less than 60 years of age, anticonvulsant discontinuation/withdrawal and low antiepileptic drug levels are the most common cause of seizures. Alcohol-related seizures account for most seizures between the ages of 30 and 60 years and are the second most common cause of seizures overall in adults. Other common causes of seizures are drug overdose, metabolic disorders, CNS infections, and trauma. Hypoglycemia and hyponatremia are the most common metabolic disorders.

The first step in the evaluation of a seizure is to determine if the event is truly a seizure. The physician should attempt to obtain a moment-by-moment description of the event from a witness. When unable to obtain a reliable history, the examining physician should assume that the seizure is a first-time event and proceed with a new-onset seizure work-up. Special consideration should be given to the possibility of toxic exposure or underlying complicating medical conditions such as alcoholism, diabetes, and renal failure. The second step is to identify possible acute precipitants for seizures. Seizures may be the manifestation of an underlying medical illness requiring specific treatment.

Medications Associated with Seizure

Amantadine

Bupropion

Carbamazepine

Citalopram

Cyclic antidepressants

Diphenhydramine

Disopyramide

Fluoride

Hydroxychloroquine

Iron

Isoniazid

Lidocaine

Lithium

Meperidine

Olanzapine

Phenytoin

Procainamide

Propoxyphene

Quinidine

Quinine

Salicylates

Selective serotonin reuptake inhibitors

Theophylline

Thioridazine

Tramadol

Venlafaxine

Causes of Seizure

Boric acid ingestion

Brain tumor

- Brain metastases
- CNS lymphoma
- Malignant glioma
- Meningiomas

Caffeine

Camphor

Carbamates

Carbon monoxide exposure

Cerebrovascular accident or transient ischemic attack

CNS infection

- Abscess
- AIDS dementia
- Bacterial meningitis
- Cryptococcal meningitis
- Cysticercosis
- Encephalitis, especially herpes
- Tuberculous meningitis

Cyanide

Degenerative disorders

- Alzheimer's dementia
- Amyloid angiopathy

Dialysis disequilibrium

Dialysis encephalopathy

Drugs of abuse

- Amphetamines
- Cocaine
- Gamma-hydroxybutyric acid
- N-methyl-D-aspartate (NMDA)
- Nicotine
- Phencyclidine

Elapid envenomation

Encephalopathy

Ephedra

Granulomatous angiitis of the CNS

Gyromitra esculenta mushroom

Head trauma

Heavy metal poisoning

- Arsenic
- Lead
- Thallium
- Hydrogen sulfide
- Hypertensive encephalopathy
- Metabolic causes
- Hyperglycemia
- Hypoglycemia
- Hyponatremia
- Hypoxia
- Uremia

Multiple sclerosis

Organochlorine pesticides

- Dichlorodiphenyltrichloroethane (DDT)
- Lindane

Organophosphates

Polyarteritis nodosa

Porphyria

Rodenticides

- Bromethalin
- Zinc phosphide

Scorpion envenomation

Sickle cell anemia

Subdural hematoma

Systemic lupus erythematosus

Thrombotic thrombocytopenia purpura

Thujone

Water hemlock

Wegener's granulomatosis

Withdrawal syndromes

- Alcohol
- Baclofen
- Sedative–hypnotic

Conditions that may mimic seizures (Table 1 in Schachter)

- Breath-holding spells
- Cardiac arrhythmia
- Conversion disorders
- Dementia
- Disassociation
- Episodic dyscontrol syndrome
- Fugue state
- Hyperventilation
- Malingering
- Migraine
- Movement disorders such as tics or Tourette's syndrome
- Panic attacks
- Paroxysmal ataxia
- Paroxysmal vertigo
- Paroxysmal kinesogenic choreoathetosis
- Periodic paralysis
- Pseudoseizure
- Psychosis
- Sleep disorders (narcolepsy, sleep paralysis)
- Somatization

- Startle syndrome
- Syncope
- Transient global amnesia

Key Historical Features

✓ Description of the event

✓ Pain or injury from the seizure

✓ Risk factors for seizure (head trauma, cerebrovascular disease)

✓ Fever

✓ Infectious symptoms

✓ Headache

✓ Complaints of focal neurologic deficits

✓ Previous seizure history

✓ Past medical history, especially diabetes, cancer, cardiac and vascular diseases, renal failure, hepatic failure, and bleeding disorders or coagulopathies

✓ Pregnancy

✓ Medications, including over-the-counter agents

✓ Alcohol and substance abuse

✓ Toxin exposure

✓ HIV risk factors

✓ Thorough review of systems

✓ Evidence of sleep disorders

Key Physical Findings

✓ Vitals signs, including presence of fever

✓ Evaluation of level of consciousness and mental status

✓ Evaluation for injuries preceding or suffered during the seizure

✓ Funduscopic examination

✓ Neck examination for nuchal rigidity

✓ Thorough neurologic examination

✓ Thorough examination for evidence of underlying systemic disease, infection, or toxic exposure

Suggested Work-Up

Complete blood count	To evaluate for evidence of infection or platelet disorder
Electrolytes	To evaluate for hyponatremia
BUN and creatinine	To evaluate for uremia
Glucose level	To evaluate for hypoglycemia or hyperglycemia
Calcium	To evaluate for calcium disturbance
Magnesium	To evaluate for magnesium disturbance
Phosphorus	To evaluate for phosphorus disturbance
ESR	To evaluate for inflammatory disorder or vasculitis
Liver function tests	To evaluate for liver disease
Electrocardiogram	May be helpful in diagnosing long QT syndrome presenting as a seizure
	A seizure with a widened QRS interval on electrocardiogram may be a clue to cyclic antidepressants, propoxyphene, venlafaxine, diphenhydramine, or other agents
Chest x-ray	Rarely adds to the discover of seizure etiology but can indicate a need for further work-up (such as malignancy)
Electroencephalogram	To help establish the diagnosis of epilepsy and classify the seizure type
Head CT or MRI	Should be performed for all first-time seizures
	CT imaging is also indicated for any patient taking anticoagulants or having coagulopathy/platelet disorders, recent head trauma, HIV-positive status or immunosuppression, history of cancer, history of alcoholism, signs of recent trauma, fever, persistent headache, or nuchal rigidity.

MRI is the neurodiagnostic study of choice when available because of its increased sensitivity for infarcts and focal gliosis.

Additional Work-Up

Echocardiogram, carotid Doppler ultrasonography, Holter monitoring	Often indicated in the patient with suspected cardiogenic syncope, transient ischemic attack, or stroke
Serum drug levels	If the patient is taking anticonvulsant medications
Toxicology screen and alcohol level	If substance abuse is suspected or the patient's mental status is not returning to normal following a seizure
Lumbar puncture	Indicated if the patient is febrile or recently febrile, is immunocompromised, or meningitis is suspected. Also indicated in patients in whom subarachnoid hemorrhage is suspected after a negative CT is obtained. May also be indicated if a clear precipitant is not found on initial evaluation
CSF fluid for herpes simplex polymerase chain reaction (PCR)	If encephalitis is suspected
Creatine kinase and troponin	In patients with known or suspected heart disease to help rule out a myocardial ischemia-induced arrhythmia
Blood alcohol level and prothrombin time	For the evaluation of an alcoholic patient
Prothrombin time and activated partial thromboplastin time	For patients taking anticoagulants or with known coagulopathies or platelet disorders
Pregnancy test	If pregnancy is suspected in a woman of childbearing age
HIV testing	If HIV infection is suspected
Blood cultures	If bacterial meningitis is suspected
Inpatient monitoring	May be indicated if the diagnosis is uncertain

Further reading

Bradford JC, Kyriakedes CG. Evaluation of the patient with seizures: an evidence based approach. Emergency Medicine Clinics of North America 1999;17: 203–220.

Roth HL, Drislane FW. Seizures. Neurologic Clinics 1998;16: 257–284.

Schachter SC. Seizure disorders. Primary Care: Clinics in Office Practice 2004;31: 85–94.

Velez L, Selwa LM. Seizure disorders in the elderly. American Family Physician 2003; 67: 325–332.

Willmore LJ. Epilepsy emergencies: the first seizure and status epilepticus. Neurology 1998;51: S034–S038.

Wills B, Erickson T. Drug- and toxin-associated seizures. Medical Clinics of North America 2005;89: 1297–1321.

63 SOLITARY PULMONARY NODULE

General Discussion

A solitary pulmonary nodule is radiologically defined as an intraparenchymal lung lesion that is less than 3 cm in diameter and is not associated with atelectasis or adenopathy. Lung lesions greater than 3 cm in diameter are defined as lung masses. Approximately one in 500 chest radiographs demonstrates a lung nodule, most of which are incidental findings. The incidence of cancer in patients with solitary nodules ranges from 10 to 70%. Infectious granulomas cause about 80% of the benign lesions, and hamartomas about 10%. Factors that increase the probability that a solitary pulmonary nodule is malignant include older age, a history of cigarette smoking, and a previous history of malignancy.

Certain radiologic characteristics also influence the probability of malignancy. The size of a lung nodule correlates with the likelihood of malignancy. The majority of lung nodules greater than 2 cm in size are malignant, while 50% of nodules less than 2 cm are malignant. Two patterns of the margins of a nodule suggest cancer. The first is the corona radiate sign, consisting of very fine linear strands extending 4 to 5 mm outward from the nodule. These have a spiculated appearance on plain radiographs. The second potentially concerning pattern is a scalloped border, which is associated with an intermediate probability of cancer. A smooth border is more suggestive of a benign diagnosis. Likewise, if benign-appearing central calcifications are seen within the solitary pulmonary nodule, further diagnostic testing usually is not indicated. Calcification patterns that are stippled or eccentric may be suggestive of malignancy and warrant further evaluation.

If a solitary pulmonary nodule is found on chest X-ray, all previous chest X-rays should be reviewed. A solitary pulmonary nodule that is unchanged on chest X-ray for at least 2 years traditionally has been considered a sign that a lesion is benign and does not require further diagnostic evaluation. However, this 2-year rule has been questioned and should be used with caution. High-resolution CT has a much better resolution, so it is probably reasonable to use 2-year stability on high-resolution CT as a practical guideline for predicting a benign process.

The growth rate of a nodule can be estimated if previous images are available. The volume-doubling time for malignant bronchogenic tumors typically is 1 to 12 months. A 30% increase in diameter represents a doubling of volume. If a lesion doubles in less than 1 month or if a nodule was not present on a radiograph obtained less than 2 months before the current image it is not likely to be malignant.

The optimal frequency of follow-up imaging is not known. However, imaging with high-resolution CT at 3-month intervals during the first year a nodule is discovered and then at 6-month intervals during the next year is an acceptable practice.

Spiral CT with intravenous contrast enhancement is the imaging modality of choice for the solitary pulmonary nodule and should be obtained on all newly diagnosed solitary pulmonary nodules. In addition to characterizing the nodule, the CT can also be used to identify other lung lesions, metastatic disease, or lymphadenopathy.

In a patient with a new finding of a solitary pulmonary nodule and a recent history of pneumonia or pulmonary symptoms, the lesion may be followed for 4–6 weeks to rule out an infectious etiology. If the nodule persists, further diagnostic evaluation is indicated.

Positron emission tomography (PET) with 18-fluorodeoxyglucose (FDG) is a very good and increasingly widely used mode of tumor imaging. Increased activity is demonstrated in cells with high metabolic rates, as is seen in tumors and areas of inflammation. PET may also provide staging information.

For operable patients with a solitary pulmonary nodule who decline surgical intervention, transthoracic needle aspiration or transbronchial needle biopsy is the preferred procedure for establishing a diagnosis. For patients with a solitary pulmonary nodule who are not operable candidates or are at high risk, transthoracic needle aspiration may be helpful to establish tissue diagnosis. Bronchoscopy often is a good approach for obtaining a tissue diagnosis for a large central lung mass or in those with endobronchial encroachment. There is little role for bronchoscopy in the patient with a peripheral lung nodule.

If a solitary pulmonary nodule is new and does not have benign-appearing calcifications it should be considered to be a malignancy until proven otherwise. Surgical resection is the ideal approach, since it is both diagnostic and therapeutic.

Suggested Work-Up

Although determining the probability of cancer in patients with solitary pulmonary nodules remains an inexact science, the pretest probability of cancer determines the strategy for the diagnosis of a solitary nodule. When the probability of cancer is low (<10%), the preferred strategy is radiographic follow-up with high-resolution CT at 3, 6, 9, 12, 18, and 24 months. When the probability is intermediate (12 to 60%), options include PET if the nodule is at least 1 cm in diameter, contrast-enhanced CT, transthoracic fine-needle aspiration biopsy if the nodule is peripherally located, or bronchoscopy. When the probability of cancer is high, surgical resection is warranted, assuming the surgical risk is acceptable.

Factors that place the patient at low risk of cancer include a nodule <1.5 cm in diameter, smooth nodule margins, patient age less than 45 years, no smoking history or having quit more than 7 years ago.

Factors that place the patient at intermediate risk of cancer include a nodule 1.5–2.2 cm in diameter, scalloped nodule margins, patient age 45–60 years, current smoking less than one pack per day or having quit less than 7 years ago.

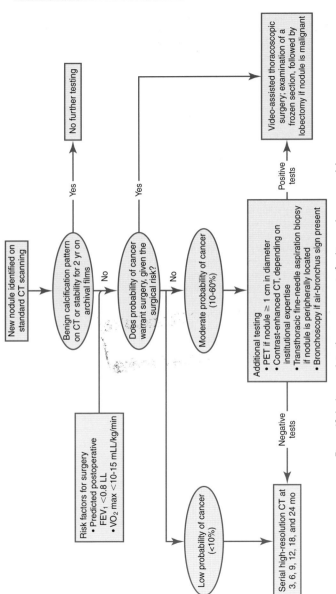

Figure 63-1. Approach to the management of solitary pulmonary nodules.

Factors that place the patient at high risk of cancer include a nodule >2.2 cm in diameter, corona radiate or spiculated nodule margins, patient age greater than 60 years, current smoking more than one pack per day and never having quit smoking.

Further reading

Lippy DM, Smith JP, Altorki NK, et al. Managing the small pulmonary nodule discovered by CT. Chest 2004;125: 1522–1529.

Ost D, Fein AM, Feinsilver SH. The solitary pulmonary nodule. New England Journal of Medicine 2003;348: 2535–2542.

Tan BB, Flaherty KR, Kazerooni EA, et al. The solitary pulmonary nodule. Chest 2003; 123: 89–96.

Yankelevitz DF, Henschke CI. Small solitary pulmonary nodules. Radiologic Clinics of North America 2000;38: 471–478.

64 SYNCOPE

General Discussion

Syncope is a sudden, unexpected loss of consciousness associated with a loss of postural tone with spontaneous recovery. A syncopal event is one of the more dramatic and anxiety-provoking symptoms encountered by patients, and often produces a diagnostic dilemma for the clinician. However, syncope is a common manifestation of numerous disorders with a final common pathway of insufficient cerebral blood flow to maintain consciousness. Syncope must be differentiated from other disorders of altered consciousness, including seizures, sleep disorders, metabolic disorders, vertigo, presyncope, and psychiatric disorders.

In the evaluation of syncope, proving a specific diagnosis is often difficult due to a lack of residual abnormalities on examination or on initial diagnostic studies. The clinician must remember that syncope is a symptom, and not a disease. By possessing an understanding of the common etiologies which cause syncope, the clinician can focus the history, physical examination, and diagnostic evaluation in each specific case. An understanding of the available diagnostic tests and their indications is imperative.

The differential diagnosis of syncope is broad, and prevalence varies depending upon research methods employed in each study. The most common causes of syncope are vasovagal syncope, arrhythmias, and orthostatic hypotension. One should remember that as many as half of patients have syncope of unknown cause after a standard diagnostic evaluation.

Many algorithms exist for the evaluation of syncope, and most emphasize the importance of the history and physical examination in making an accurate diagnosis. A position paper published by the American College of Physicians presents the following important features in guiding diagnosis:

- Separate patients into diagnostic, suggestive, and unexplained categories on the basis of the history, physical examination, and ECG findings.
- Separate patients with unexplained syncope further on the basis of age and the presence of organic heart disease or an abnormal ECG.
- Use echocardiography and treadmill stress testing to evaluate and quantify the degree of heart disease
- Reserve Holter monitoring and electrophysiology studies for patients with confirmed heart disease.
- Employ tilt testing, loop recorders, and psychiatric evaluation in patients with recurrent unexplained syncope and no suspected heart disease or a negative cardiac evaluation.

Although algorithms may provide a guide for the evaluation of syncope, the various available algorithms each contain controversial elements. In addition, algorithms do not consider every clinical situation and are not designed to replace individual clinician judgment. The physician should understand the approach to the patient with syncope first, and then consult algorithms to focus the diagnostic evaluation.

Medications Associated with Syncope

Alpha-agonists

Anticholinergic agents

Antiparkinsonian agents

Antipsychotics

Beta-adrenergic blockers

Narcotics

Vasodilators

Causes of Syncope

Reflex mediated

- Vasovagal
- Situational (cough, defecation, micturition, swallow)
- Carotid sinus hypersensitivity

Cardiac

- Arrhythmia
- Hypertrophic cardiomyopathy
- Tamponade
- Valvular disease

Medication effects

Metabolic disorders

- Adrenal failure

Hypoglycemia

Neurologic causes

- Migraine headache
- Transient ischemic attack

Orthostatic hypotension (autonomic dysfunction)

- Diabetes
- Amyloidosis
- Paraneoplastic neuropathies
- HIV infection
- Guillain–Barré syndrome

- Parkinson's disease
- Shy–Drager syndrome

Psychiatric causes

- Major depression
- Panic disorder
- Pseudoseizures

Other causes

- Hypovolemia
- Hyperventilation
- Seizure (not a true case of syncope)
- Subclavian steal syndrome

Unknown

Key Historical Features

✓ Situation in which syncope occurred (upon standing, in a fearful situation, during micturition, with coughing, with exertion)

✓ Prodromal symptoms (lightheadedness, warmth, nausea, sweating)

✓ Associated cardiac symptoms (chest pain, palpitations, shortness of breath)

✓ Associated neurologic symptoms (focal neurologic symptoms, headache, diplopia)

✓ Witnessed events (tonic/clonic movements, tongue biting, urinary incontinence)

✓ Previous history of syncope

✓ Recent dehydration

✓ Postevent symptoms

- Confusion may indicate seizure activity
- Injuries related to a fall
- Duration of recovery

✓ Past medical history, particularly:

- History of cardiac disease, including coronary artery disease, arrhythmias, or cardiomyopathy
- History of cerebrovascular ischemia
- History of pulmonary embolism or pulmonary hypertension
- History of gastrointestinal bleeding

✓ Family history of syncope or sudden death

✓   Medications

- Especially antihypertensive agents, antidepressants, vasodilators, narcotic analgesics, Q-T prolonging agents (tricyclic antidepressants), and hypoglycemic agents

✓   Social history

- Alcohol or marijuana use
- Smoking history which places the patient at risk for cardiopulmonary disease

Key Physical Findings

✓   Vitals signs

✓   Evaluation for orthostatic hypotension (defined as at least a 20 mm Hg systolic or 10 mm Hg diastolic blood pressure within 3 minutes of standing)

✓   Cardiovascular examination

- Carotid bruits
- Murmurs
- Jugular venous distention
- Loud S2
- Presence of an S3
- Pericardial friction rubs
- Blood pressures in both the arms

✓   Neurologic evaluation

- Mental status
- Pupil symmetry
- Evaluation for nystagmus
- Gait
- Balance

Suggested Work-Up

CBC, electrolytes, BUN, creatinine, and glucose	Indicated when an underlying disorder is suspected as a potential cause of syncope
Pregnancy test	Should be considered in women of childbearing age

Electrocardiogram	To identify abnormalities that may suggest an underlying cardiac cause for the syncope. Important findings include evidence of conduction disorders, signs of coronary artery disease, or left ventricular hypertrophy that may be associated with ventricular tachycardia
Holter monitoring or telemetry monitoring	Recommended for patients with known or suspected cardiac disease or a suspected arrhythmic cause of syncope

Additional Work-Up

Tilt table testing	May be useful in patients with recurrent unexplained syncope with a suspected neurocardiogenic cause. May also be useful in patients without cardiac disease or in whom cardiac testing has been negative
Echocardiography	To rule out a cardiac cause of syncope in patients with suspected cardiac disease. In patients with exertional syncope, echocardiography can help exclude hypertrophic cardiomyopathy and aortic stenosis
Exercise tolerance testing	To confirm and quantify coronary artery disease in patients with syncope in whom coronary artery disease is suspected. Exercise tolerance testing also may be used to rule out coronary artery disease and exercise-induced arrhythmias in patients with exertional syncope
Electrophysiology study	To diagnose conduction disease or susceptibility for developing tachyarrhythmias in patients with a suspected arrhythmic cause for their syncope and a history of known heart disease, especially previous myocardial infarction or congestive heart failure. May also be used for patients with preexcitation syndromes such as Wolff–Parkinson–White syndrome and in patients with a suspected bradyarrhythmic cause for syncope, particularly older patients

Transtelephonic electrocardiogram monitoring	Most useful in patients with frequent syncope and either no suspected cardiac disease or a negative cardiac evaluation
Insertable loop recorder	May be useful in patients without evidence of neurocardiogenic syncope or organic heart disease and with infrequent episodes of syncope that make the use of an external loop recorder impractical
EEG	The diagnostic yield of EEG is very low and is indicated only when seizure is suspected
CT	CT scanning of the head has a relatively low yield in patients with syncope and is not routinely indicated. It is recommended in patients with focal neurologic symptoms and signs. It may be performed in patients with seizure activity and head trauma to rule out intracranial hemorrhage
Vascular studies	Carotid ultrasonography or transcranial Doppler add little in the evaluation of syncope. Carotid disease or vertebrobasilar disease significant enough to cause a loss of consciousness would be unlikely in the absence of other neurologic signs such as diplopia, dysarthria, or vertigo
Carotid sinus massage	May be considered in selected patients 60 years or older with an otherwise nondiagnostic evaluation for syncope
Psychiatric evaluation	Recommended for patients with recurrent unexplained syncope if there is no cardiac disease or if the cardiac evaluation is negative. Young patients and patients with many prodromal symptoms are at higher risk of having an underlying psychiatric disease associated with their episodes of syncope

Further reading

Abboud FM. Neurocardiogenic syncope. New England Journal of Medicine 1993;328: 1117–1120.

Atkins D, Hanusa B, Sefcik T, et al. Syncope and orthostatic hypotension. American Journal of Medicine 1991;91: 179–185.

Calkins H. Pharmacologic approaches to therapy for vasovagal syncope. American Journal of Cardiology 1999;84: 20Q–25Q.

Cunningham R, Mikhail MG. Management of patients with syncope and cardiac arrhythmias in an emergency department observation unit. Emergency Medicine Clinics of North America 2001;19: 105–121.

Davis TL, Freemon FR. Electroencephalography should not be routine in the evaluation of syncope in adults. Archives of Internal Medicine 1990;150: 2027–2029.

Di Girolamo E, Di Iorio C, Sabatini P, et al. Effects of paroxetine hydrochloride, a selective serotonin reuptake inhibitor, on refractory vasovagal syncope: A randomized, double-blind, placebo-controlled study. Johurnal of the American College of Cardiology 1999; 33: 1227–1230.

Kapoor WN. Syncope. New England Journal of Medicine 2000;343: 1856–1862.

Kaufmann H. Neurally mediated syncope: pathogenesis, diagnosis, and treatment. Neurology 1995;45(Suppl 5): S12–S18.

Linzer M, Yang EH, Estes 3rd NA, et al. Diagnosing syncope: Part 1: Value of history, physical examination and electrocardiography. Clinical efficacy assessment project of the American College of Physicians. Annals of Internal Medicine 1997;126: 989–996.

Linzer M, Yang EH, Estes 3rd NA, et al. Diagnosing syncope: Part 2. Unexplained syncope. Clinical efficacy project of the American College of Physicians. Annals of Internal Medicine 1997;127: 76–86.

Mahanonda N, Bhuripanyo K, Kangkagate C, et al. Randomized double-blind, placebo-controlled trial of oral atenolol in patients with unexplained syncope and positive upright tilt table test results. American Heart Journal 1995;130: 1250–1253.

Munro NC, McIntosh S, Lawson J, et al. Incidence of complications after carotid sinus massage in older patients with syncope. Journal of the American Geriatric Society 1994; 42: 1248–1251.

Schnipper JL, Kapoor WN. Diagnostic evaluation and management of patients with syncope. Medical Clinics of North America 2001;85: 423–456.

Sutton R, Brignole M, Menozzi C, et al. Dual chamber pacing in the treatment of neurally mediated positive cardioinhibitory syncope: pacemaker versus no therapy – a multicenter randomized study. The Vasovagal Syncope International Study (VASIS) investigators. Circulation 2000;102: 294–299.

Sutton R, Petersen M, Brignole M, et al. Proposed classification for tilt induced vasovagal syncope. European Journal of Pacing Electrophysiology 1992;3: 180–183.

Ward CR, Gray JC, Gilroy JJ, et al. Midodrine: A role in the management of neurocardiogenic syncope. Heart 1998;79: 45–49.

Weimer LH. Syncope and orthostatic intolerance for the primary care physician. Primary Care Clinics in Office Practice 2004;31: 175–199.

Zeng C, Zhu Z, Liu G, et al. Randomized, double-blind, placebo-controlled trial of oral enalapril in patients with neurally mediated syncope. American Heart Journal 1998;136: 852–858.

Zimetbaum P, Kim KY, Ho KK, et al. Utility of patient-activated cardiac event recorders in general clinical practice. American Journal of Cardiology 1997;79: 371–372.

General Discussion

Analysis of synovial fluid plays a major role in the diagnosis of joint disease. Several classification schemes have been used to help classify joint diseases. When using classification schemes, it is important to realize that considerable overlap may occur in synovial fluid findings among different groups. In addition, more than one diagnosis may be present, such as a septic joint in a patient with rheumatoid arthritis. Findings on synovial fluid analysis may be classified as normal, noninflammatory, inflammatory, infectious, crystal-associated, and hemorrhagic.

Routine examination of synovial fluid should include: (1) gross examination of color and clarity; (2) total leukocyte and differential counts; (3) Gram's stain and bacterial culture, both aerobic and anaerobic; and (4) crystal examination with polarizing microscopy.

Additional studies may be indicated under certain circumstances and should be guided by clinical suspicion. These studies include fungal and acid-fast stains and cultures, countercurrent immunoelectrophoresis for bacterial antigens, lactate levels, complement levels, and the presence of certain enzymes such as lactate dehydrogenase.

Suggested Work-Up

See Table 65.1 below for the interpretation of findings.
Physical characteristics of the fluid

- Color
- Clarity
- Viscosity

Microscopic appearance

- WBC count and differential
- Crystals (polarized light)

Microbiology

- Gram's stain
- Bacterial culture (aerobic and anaerobic)

Additional Work-Up

| Fungal culture | To evaluate for fungal arthritis when it is suspected |
| Culture for *Mycobacterium tuberculosis* | To evaluate for tuberculous arthritis when it is suspected |

Classification	Appearance	WBCs/µL	PMNs (%)	Crystals	Culture
Normal	Clear to straw-colored	<150	<25	No	Negative
Noninflammatory Osteoarthritis Traumatic arthritis Neuroarthropathy Early RA Paget's disease Acromegaly Hyperparathyroidism	Yellow, transparent	<3000	<30	No	Negative
Inflammatory RA Lupus erythematosus Scleroderma Reiter's syndrome Ankylosing spondylitis Rheumatic fever Ulcerative colitis Sarcoidosis Polymyalgia rheumatica	Yellow, cloudy, or bloody	3000–75 000	>50	No	Negative
Infectious Bacterial Mycobacterial Fungal Viral Spirochetal	Yellow, purulent	50 000–200 000	>90	No	Often positive
Crystal-induced Gout CPPD	Cloudy, turbid	500–200 000	<90	Yes	Negative
Hemorrhagic Traumatic arthritis Hemophiliac arthropathy Anticoagulation Thrombocytopenia	Red–brown	50–10 000	<50	No	Negative

Abbreviations: CPPD, calcium pyrophosphate dihydrate; RA, rheumatoid arthritis.

Table 65-1. Classification of Synovial Fluid

Serum and synovial fluid glucose levels	A serum-synovia differential is less than 10 mg/dL in normal fluid and many noninflammatory conditions. In septic arthritis, the differential ranges from 20 to 60 mg/dL but overlaps with other inflammatory conditions
Serum and synovial fluid complement levels	Complement levels in synovial fluid normally are about 10% of serum levels. Inflammatory conditions increases this to 40–70% of serum levels

Further reading

Henry JB. Cerebrospinal, synovial, and serous body fluids. In: Clinical diagnosis and management by laboratory methods. Philadelphia: Saunders; 1996:467–472.

Kjeldsberg CR, Knight JA. Body fluids: laboratory examinations of amniotic, cerebrospinal, seminal, serous and synovial fluids, 3rd ed. Chicago: American Society of Clinical Pathologists.

O'Connell TX. Interpreting tests from joint aspirates. Atlas Office Procedures 2000;5: 423–431.

Schmerling RH, et al. Synovial fluid tests-What should be ordered? Journal of the American Medical Association 1990;260: 1009.

Schumacher HR. Synovial fluid analysis and synovial biopsy. In: Textbook of rheumatology, 4th ed. Philadelphia: Saunders; 1993: 562–570.

Tierney LM, McPhee SJ, Papadakis MA. Arthritis and musculoskeletal disorders. In: Current medical diagnosis and treatment. New York: Lange; 2000:807–808.

General Discussion

When evaluating a scrotal mass, it should be classified as extratesticular or intratesticular, solid or cystic, and painless or painful. Masses which arise from the testicle are more likely to represent malignancies, while extratesticular masses are more likely to be benign. Likewise, solid masses are much more likely to represent neoplastic conditions, especially when painless. Transillumination using a hand-held light source may help differentiate between solid and cystic structures. Extratesticular tumors are uncommon but do occur in the form of para-testicular rhabdomyosarcoma or adenomatoid tumors of the epididymis.

Cystic lesions of the scrotum are much more common than solid lesions. A cystic mass within the epididymis is usually a spermatocele. A cyst within the spermatic cord usually represents a hydrocele. A cystic mass that surrounds the entire testicle usually represents a hydrocele.

Although a careful physical examination may be diagnostic, confirmation using scrotal ultrasonography is recommended to confirm the location of the mass and to differentiate between solid and cystic lesions.

A testicular tumor usually presents as a painless mass, though the patient may complain of scrotal heaviness or a dull ache. If testicular cancer is suspected, the patient should also be examined for lymphadenopathy, gynecomastia, and abdominal masses.

A hydrocele is a collection of peritoneal fluid between the layers of the tunica vaginalis surrounding the testicle. A hydrocele usually presents as a painless scrotal swelling that can be transilluminated. The swelling often worsens during the course of the day, and the patient may complain of weight and bulk as a result of the hydrocele. A new hydrocele or one that hemorrhages as a result of minor trauma may indicate an underlying testicular cancer.

A spermatocele usually presents as a painless cystic mass superior and posterior to the testis. This mass is separate from the testis, is freely mobile, and transilluminates easily.

A varicocele is present in up to 20% of all males and is a tortuous and dilated pampiniform venous plexus and internal spermatic vein. Varicoceles often are described as a "bag of worms" superior to, and distinct from, the testicle. Varicoceles usually first appear near mid-puberty. Most varicoceles occur on the left side and often are asymptomatic, though they may cause male infertility. The dilatation and tortuosity are most noticeable when the patient is upright, and may be accentuated if the patient performs a Valsalva maneuver.

Causes of Testicular Masses

Acute orchitis

Epididymitis

Hydrocele

Inguinal hernia

Spermatocele

Testicular cancer

Testicular torsion with associated swelling

Key Historical Features

✓   Duration of the mass

✓   Pain

✓   Constitutional symptoms such as weight loss, fever, chest pain, cough, headache

✓   Past medical history

✓   Past surgical history

✓   Family history

Key Physical Findings

✓   Careful palpation and identification of the intrascrotal contents

✓   Testicular examination for volume, masses, or tenderness

✓   Transillumination of the testicular mass

✓   Palpation of the epididymis

✓   Assessment of the spermatic cord

✓   Cremasteric reflex

✓   Examination of the inguinal canals for a hernia or cord tenderness

✓   Valsalva maneuver to evaluate for hernia or varicocele

✓   Abdominal examination for masses

✓   Breast examination for gynecomastia

✓   Lymph node examination

Suggested Work-Up

Scrotal ultrasound	To help define suspected lesions and differentiate between intratesticular and extratesticular lesions

Additional Work-Up

Serum alpha fetoprotein (AFP)	If testicular cancer is suspected. Elevated AFP level implies nonseminomatous germ cell tumor or mixed tumor
Serum human chorionic gonadotropin (HCG)	If testicular cancer is suspected. HCG is secreted by one-half of nonseminomatous germ cell tumors and mixed tumors as well as 10% of pure seminomas
Lactate dehydrogenase	If testicular cancer is suspected. Lactate dehydrogenase is elevated in 60% of nonseminomatous germ cell tumors
Abdominal CT scan, chest x-ray, and CT scan of the lungs	Performed for staging purposes if a testicular malignancy is identified

Further reading

Haynes, JH. Inguinal and scrotal disorders. Surgical Clinics of North America 2006;86: 371–381.

Jayanthi VR. Adolescent urology. Adolescent Medicine Clinics 2004;15: 521–534.

Junnila J, Lassen P. Testicular masses. American Family Physician 1998;57: 685–692.

General Discussion

Thrombocytopenia is defined as a platelet count below the normal range for the population, which is between 150 000 and 450 000/μL. Healthy women may experience mild to moderate thrombocytopenia in the range of 75 000–150 000/μL during pregnancy and do not require any investigation.

The diagnostic evaluation of thrombocytopenia begins by excluding artifactual or pseudothrombocytopenia as the etiology. This is caused by platelet clumping when EDTA is used as an anticoagulant in the blood sample. The presence of platelet clumps on examination of the peripheral smear and a normal repeat platelet count using citrated blood confirms pseudothrombocytopenia as the cause.

After pseudothrombocytopenia has been excluded, the possibility of thrombotic thrombocytopenic purpura/hemolytic uremic syndrome (TTP/HUS) should be considered. A peripheral blood smear with schistocytes, increased serum levels of lactate dehydrogenase (LDH), and decreased serum haptoglobin suggest TTP/HUS or disseminated intravascular coagulation (DIC). Coagulation studies are usually normal in TTP/HUS but are prolonged in DIC.

Once TTP/HUS and DIC have been excluded, drug-related thrombocytopenia and hypersplenism should be considered as possible causes. If heparin-induced thrombocytopenia is considered, the diagnosis may be confirmed by in vitro testing to detect heparin-dependent platelet antibodies.

Idiopathic thrombocytopenic purpura (ITP) is a diagnosis of exclusion. Other causes of immune-mediated thrombocytopenia should be considered. These include connective tissue disease, lymphoproliferative disorders, and HIV infection.

Medications Associated with Thrombocytopenia

Abciximab

Acetaminophen

Aminoglutethimide

Aminosalicylic acid

Amiodarone

Amphotericin B

Ampicillin

Amrinone

Captopril

Carbamazepine

Chlorothiazide

Chlorpromazine

Chlorpropamide

Cimetidine

Cisplatin

Clopidogrel

Cyclosporine A

Danazol

Deferoxamine

Diatrizoate meglumine

Diazepam

Diazoxide

Diclofenac

Diethylstilbestrol

Digoxin

Eptifibatide

Furosemide

Gold

Haloperidol

Heparin

Hydrochlorothiazide

Ibuprofen

Interferon alpha

Isoniazid

Levamisole

Lithium

Meclofenamate

Methicillin

Methyldopa

Minoxidil

Mitomycin A

Nalidixic acid

Naphazoline

Oxyphenbutazone

Oxytetracycline

Phenytoin

Piperacillin

Procainamide

Quinidine

Quinine

Ranitidine

Rifampin

Sulfasalazine

Sulfisoxazole

Sulindac

Tamoxifen

Thiothixene

Ticlopidine

Tirofiban

Trimethoprim/sulfamethoxazole

Valproic acid

Vancomycin

Causes of Thrombocytopenia

Amegakaryocytic thrombocytopenia

Antiphospholipid syndrome

Aplastic anemia

Bernard–Soulier syndrome

Bone marrow transplantation

Cardiac bypass

Cardiac valves

Common variable hypogammaglobulinemia

Connective tissue diseases

Disseminated intravascular coagulation

Escherichia coli O157:H7 infection

Epstein–Barr virus

Gray platelet syndrome

HELLP syndrome

Hematologic malignancies

Hemolytic uremic syndrome

Heparin-induced thrombocytopenia

Hepatitis C infection

Hereditary thrombocytopenias

HIV infection

Hypersplenism

ITP

IgA deficiency

Kasabach–Merritt syndrome

May–Hegglin anomaly

Medications

Metastatic cancer to bone marrow

Myelodysplastic syndrome

Paroxysmal nocturnal hemoglobinuria

Post transfusion purpura

Pregnancy

Primary bone marrow disorder

Radiation

Rheumatoid arthritis

Sepsis

Systemic lupus erythematosus

Thrombotic thrombocytopenic purpura

Vitamin D deficiency

X-linked Wiskott–Aldrich syndrome

Key Historical Features

✓ Easy bruising

✓ Gingival bleeding

✓ Epistaxis

✓ Menorrhagia

✓ Gastrointestinal bleeding

✓ Recent respiratory illness

✓ Past medical history, especially a history of low platelet counts or bleeding tendency

✓ Medications

✓ Use of over-the-counter products

✓ Family history of platelet disorders or bleeding tendency

✓ Alcohol consumption

✓ HIV risk factors

Key Physical Findings

✓   Vital signs

✓   Head and neck examination for evidence of bleeding in the mucous membranes

✓   Funduscopic examination for evidence of retinal hemorrhage

✓   Lymphadenopathy

✓   Evidence of bleeding in the skin

✓   Cardiac examination for tachycardia

✓   Abdominal examination for splenomegaly

✓   Rectal examination including stool hemoccult testing to evaluate for gastrointestinal bleeding

✓   Neurologic examination to help evaluate for intracranial bleed

Suggested Work-Up

Peripheral blood smear	To evaluate for schistocytes (hemolysis)
Serum lactate dehydrogenase	Increased in hemolysis
Serum haptoglobin	Decreased in hemolysis
PT, PTT, fibrin split products, fibrinogen, D-dimer	To evaluate for disseminated intravascular coagulation

Additional Work-Up

Coombs test	If hemolysis is suspected
HIV, antinuclear antibodies, and serum protein electrophoresis	Should be ordered before ITP is diagnosed to evaluate for HIV infection, autoimmune disease, and lymphoproliferative disease
Vitamin B_{12} and folate levels	If nutritional causes of thrombocytopenia are suspected
Bone marrow examination	Indicated when a platelet production problem is suspected. In elderly patients, patients with abnormalities in red and/or white cells, and in patients without a definitive cause after initial work-up, a bone marrow biopsy may elucidate the presence of a primary marrow disorder

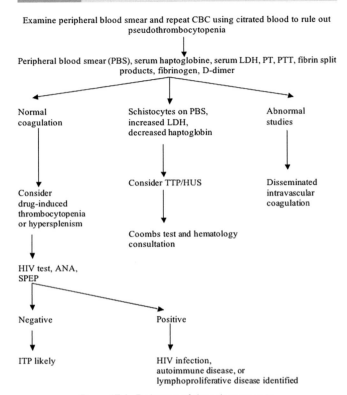

Figure 67-1. Evaluation of thrombocytopenia.

Further reading

Cines DB, Blanchette VS. Immune thrombocytopenic purpura. New England Journal of Medicine 2002;346(13): 995–1008.

Sekhon SS, Roy V. Thrombocytopenia in adults: a practical approach to evaluation and management. Southern Medical Journal 2006;99: 491–498.

Tefferi A, Hanson CA, Inwards DJ. How to interpret and pursue an abnormal complete blood cell count in adults. Mayo Clinic Proceedings 2005;80(7): 923–936.

Vandendries ER, Drews RE. Drug-associated disease: hematologic dysfunction. Critical Care Clinics 2006;22: 347–355.

General Discussion

The prevalence of palpable thyroid nodules is 3–7% in North America. Thyroid nodules are more common in elderly persons, in women, in those with iodine deficiency, and in those with a history of radiation exposure. The clinical importance of thyroid nodules is primarily the need to exclude the presence of a malignant thyroid lesion, which accounts for about 5% of all thyroid nodules, regardless of the size of the nodule.

Characteristics that may increase the risk of thyroid cancer include a history of prior head and neck irradiation, a family history of medullary thyroid carcinoma or multiple endocrine neoplasia type 2, age less than 20 years or greater than 70 years, male gender, a growing nodule, a firm nodule, cervical lymphadenopathy, a fixed nodule, dysphonia, dysphagia, or cough.

Key Historical Features

✓ Age

✓ Gender

✓ Symptoms of hypo- or hyperthyroidism

✓ Rate of growth of the nodule

✓ Duration of the nodule

✓ Pain

✓ History of radiation to the head or neck

✓ Recent pregnancy

✓ Family history of autoimmune thyroid disease, thyroid carcinoma, multiple endocrine neoplasia, or familial polyposis

✓ Symptoms such as dysphagia, dysphonia, or hemoptysis

✓ Difficulty swallowing

Key Physical Findings

✓ Size of the nodule

✓ Fixation of the nodule to skin or soft tissue

✓ Movement of the nodule with swallowing

✓ Tenderness to palpation

✓ Presence of cervical lymphadenopathy

Suggested Work-Up

TSH	To confirm a euthyroid state or detect the presence of hypo- or hyperthyroidism
Thyroid ultrasound	For all patients with a palpable thyroid nodule to detect features suggestive of malignant growth and select the lesions to be recommended for fine needle aspiration biopsy, to look for coincidental thyroid nodules, to measure the baseline volume of the lesion, and to help choose the size of the biopsy needle
Fine needle aspiration	Recommended for most nodules, but also may be determined based upon TSH level and ultrasound findings
T3, T4, and radioisotope scan of the thyroid	If the TSH level is low to evaluate for thyrotoxicosis and to determine regional uptake or function within the thyroid gland

Additional Work-Up

CBC and ESR	If inflammatory or infectious thyroiditis is suspected
Thyroperoxidase antibody, T4, and thyroglobulin test	May be helpful in the diagnosis of Graves' disease or Hashimoto's thyroiditis when the initial TSH is elevated
Calcitonin level	Should be considered in patients with familial medullary thyroid carcinoma or multiple endocrine neoplasia

Further reading

American Association of Clinical Endocrinologists and Associazione Medici Endocrinologi Medical Guidelines for Clinical Practice for the Diagnosis and Management of Thyroid Nodules. Endocrine Practice 2006;12: 63–102.

Gharib H. Fine-needle aspiration biopsy of thyroid nodules: advantages, limitations, and effect. Mayo Clinic Proceedings 1994;69: 44–49.

Kim N, Lavertu P. Evaluation of a thyroid nodule. Otolaryngologic Clinics of North America 2003;26: 17–33.

Welker MJ, Orlov D. Thyroid nodules. American Family Physician 2003;67: 559–566.

General Discussion

Tinnitus is an unwanted auditory perception of internal origin which is usually localized and rarely heard by others. Tinnitus may affect 10–15% of the US population with the prevalence increasing with age. Other factors that may affect the prevalence of tinnitus include gender, race, socioeconomic status, hearing loss, and noise exposure.

The most accepted theory of tinnitus pathophysiology is that of outer hair cell damage, resulting in altered stiffness and thus increased discharge rates. When the discharge rate rises above the background level, tinnitus becomes troublesome. The physician's role is to determine which factors may have led to the increase in the discharge rate and which factors diminish it.

Tinnitus is often classified as either subjective or objective. Subjective tinnitus is heard only by the patient while objective tinnitus can be heard by both the patient and the examiner. Objective tinnitus usually has an identifiable acoustic source whereas subjective tinnitus is more commonly idiopathic. Tinnitus can be further classified by whether it is pulsatile or nonpulsatile and can also be graded based upon volume or severity. Unilateral or pulsatile tinnitus is more likely to represent serious underlying disease and generally warrants an evaluation by an otolaryngologist.

Medications That Can Cause Tinnitus

Aminoglycosides

Aspirin

Bumetanide

Chemotherapy agents

- Bleomycin
- Cisplatin
- Mechlorethamine
- Methotrexate
- Vincristine

Chloramphenicol

Chloroquine

Erythromycin

Ethacrynic acid

Furosemide

Heterocyclic antidepressants

NSAIDs

Quinine

Tetracycline

Vancomycin

Causes of Tinnitus

Acoustic neuroma

Arterial bruit

Arteriovenous malformation

Head injury

Hearing loss

Heavy metal exposure (mercury, lead)

Hyperlipidemia

Idiopathic stapedial muscle spasm

Lead

Medications

Menière's disease

Mercury

Multiple sclerosis

Palatomyoclonus

Patulous eustachian tube

Thyroid disorder

Vascular tumors

Venous hum

Vitamin B_{12} deficiency

Psychogenic causes

- Anxiety
- Depression
- Fibromyalgia

Key Historical Features

✓ Onset

✓ Unilateral or bilateral

✓ Pattern (continuous, episodic, pulsatile)

✓ Pitch

✓ Exacerbating and ameliorating factors

✓ Associated vertigo, hearing loss, aural fullness

✓ Presence of hearing loss

- ✓ Exposure to ototoxic medications
- ✓ Medical history, especially thyroid disorders, hyperlipidemia, vitamin B_{12} deficiency, anemia

Key Physical Findings

- ✓ Inspection of the external canal and tympanic membrane
- ✓ Cranial nerve examination
- ✓ Auscultation over the neck, periauricular area, mastoid, and orbits
- ✓ Weber and Rinne tests

Suggested Work-Up

Audiography	Helps determine need for more advanced diagnostic testing and evaluates for hearing loss
Speech discrimination testing	May help detect pathology in the CNS
Tympanometry	To help identify middle ear effusions, changes in tympanic membrane stiffness, or myoclonus of the stapedial muscle

The following should be ordered if the history and physical suggest an underlying medical abnormality:

TSH	To evaluate for thyroid disorder
Hemoglobin and hematocrit	To evaluate for anemia
Serum glucose	To evaluate for diabetes
Electrolytes, BUN, creatinine	To evaluate for metabolic derangements
Lipid panel	To evaluate for hyperlipidemia
RPR	To evaluate for neurosyphilis
Consider ESR, ANA, RF	If autoimmune disease is suspected

Additional Work-Up

MRI of the internal auditory canals	For patients with unilateral tinnitus and sensorineural hearing loss and those with asymmetric hearing loss suspicious for an acoustic neuroma
CT of the temporal bones	For patients suspected of having hereditary hearing loss, otosclerosis, Paget's disease, or trauma
Referral to an otolaryngologist	For patients with unilateral or pulsatile tinnitus

Further reading

Crummer RW, Hassan GA. Diagnostic approach to tinnitus. American Family Physician 2004;69: 120–126.

Heller AJ. Classification and epidemiology of tinnitus. Otolaryngologic Clinics of North America 2003;36: 239–248.

Lockwood AH. Tinnitus. Neurologic Clinics 2005;23: 893–900.

Meyerhoff WL, Cooper JC. Tinnitus. In: Paparella MM, ed. Otolaryngology, 3rd ed. Philadelphia: Saunders; 1991:1169–1175.

Schwaber MK. Medical evaluation of tinnitus. Otolaryngologic Clinics of North America 2003;36: 287–292.

Tyler RS. Does tinnitus originate from hyperactive nerve fibers in the cochlea? Journal of Neurophysiology 1984;44: 76–96.

General Discussion

The following discussion applies to mild elevations of liver transaminase levels (up to five times normal) in asymptomatic patients. The first step in the evaluation of the patient is to repeat the test to confirm the result. Both alanine aminotransferase (ALT) and aspartate aminotransferase (AST) are released into the blood in increasing amounts when the liver cell membrane is damaged. However, necrosis of liver cells is not required for the release of the aminotransferases, and there is a poor correlation between the level of the aminotransferases and the degree of liver cell damage.

The initial evaluation includes a detailed history, review of medications, and a physical examination. The history should include an assessment of the patient's risk factors for liver disease with attention directed toward family history, medications, vitamins, herbal supplements, alcohol consumption, drug use, history of blood-product transfusions, and symptoms of liver disease. Signs of liver disease are outlined below.

The most common causes of elevated aminotransferase levels are alcohol-related liver injury, hepatitis B and C, autoimmune hepatitis, fatty infiltration of the liver, nonalcoholic steatohepatitis (NASH), hemochromatosis, Wilson's disease, alpha$_1$-antitrypsin deficiency, and celiac sprue.

According to the American Gastroenterological Association (AGA), 1–4% of the asymptomatic population may have elevated serum liver chemistries. A minor elevation (less than twice the normal value) may be of no clinical importance if the disorders listed below have been ruled out. If the aminotransferase levels are less than twice normal and no chronic liver condition has been identified, observation alone may be indicated. If the aminotransferases are persistently more than twice normal, a liver biopsy may be indicated.

Medications That May Cause Transaminase Elevation

Acetaminophen

Amiodarone

Amoxicillin–clavulanic acid

Aspirin

Azathioprine/6-mp

Carbamazepine

Ciprofloxacin

Cyclosporine

Erythromycin

Estrogens

Fluconazole

Glipizide

Glucocorticoids

Glyburide

Halothane

Heparin

Isoniazid

Ketoconazole

L-asparaginase

Labetalol

Methotrexate

Minocycline

Nitrofurantoin

NSAIDs

Pemoline

Phenobarbital

Phenytoin

Propylthiouracil

Protease inhibitors

Statin medications

Sulfonamides

Synthetic penicillins

Trazodone

Valproic acid

Causes of Transaminitis

Acquired muscle diseases

Acute viral hepatitis

Alcohol

Alpha$_1$-antitrypsin deficiency

Autoimmune hepatitis

Celiac disease

Chronic hepatitis B

Chronic hepatitis C

Cirrhosis

Hemochromatosis

Hemolysis

Hyperthyroidism

Inherited disorders of muscle metabolism

Medications

NASH

Non-prescription medications

- Alchemilla
- Anabolic steroids
- Chaparral leaf
- Cocaine
- Ephedra (mahuang)
- Gentian
- Germander
- Glues containing toluene
- Jin bu huan
- Kava
- MDMA ("ecstasy")
- Phencyclidine
- Scutellaria (skullcap)
- Senna
- Shark cartilage
- Trichloroethylene
- Vitamin A

Steatosis

Strenuous exercise

Wilson's disease (in patients less than 40 years old)

Key Physical Findings

✓   Ascites

✓   Bleeding problems

✓   Caput medusae

✓   Gynecomastia

✓   Hemorrhoids

✓   Impotence

✓   Jaundice

✓   Liver size

- ✓ Mental status changes
- ✓ Palmar erythema
- ✓ Spider angiomata
- ✓ Splenomegaly
- ✓ Testicular atrophy

Suggested Work-Up

ALT, AST, bilirubin, alkaline	AST:ALT ratio >2 suggests alcohol abuse
Phosphatase, GGT	AST:ALT ratio <1 suggests NASH
Prothrombin time	To assess hepatic synthetic function
Albumin	To assess hepatic synthetic function
CBC	To evaluate for infection, neutropenia, thrombocytopenia
Hepatitis C antibody	To evaluate for hepatitis C
Hepatitis B surface antigen, surface antibody, and core antibody	To evaluate for hepatitis B
Serum iron, ferritin, and total iron-binding capacity	Iron overload suggests hemochromatosis
Serum ceruloplasmin	Decreased level suggests Wilson's disease
Serum protein electrophoresis	Increase in polyclonal immunoglobulins suggests autoimmune hepatitis (ANA and anti-smooth muscle antibody may be useful)
	Marked decrease in alpha-globulin bands suggests alpha$_1$-antitrypsin deficiency

Additional Work-Up (may be indicated if above tests are normal)

Quantitative hepatitis C virus RNA	If hepatitis C antibody is positive

Alpha₁-antitrypsin phenotyping	To evaluate for alpha₁-antitrypsin deficiency
Antigliadin and antiendomesial antibodies	Antibodies indicate celiac sprue
Creatine kinase and aldolase	Rule out myopathy or elevations caused by strenuous exercise
Liver ultrasonography	May reveal disorders such as hepatic steatosis and NASH
Liver biopsy	Used on a case-by-case basis

Further reading

American Gastroenterological Association. Medical position statement: evaluation of liver chemistry tests. Gastroenterology 2002;123: 1364–1366.

Giboney PT. Mildly elevated liver transaminase levels in the asymptomatic patient. American Family Physician 2005;71: 1105–1110.

Green RM, Flamm S. AGA technical review on the evaluation of liver chemistry tests. Gastroenterology 2002;123: 1367–1384.

Pratt DS, Kaplan MM. Evaluation of abnormal liver enzyme results in asymptomatic patients. New England Journal of Medicine 2000;342: 1266–1271.

Swartz MH. Textbook of physical diagnosis, 2nd ed. Philadelphia: Saunders; 1994:302–336.

General Discussion

The first step in evaluating any patient with tremor is to characterize the tremor. All humans have physiologic tremor of the hands which may be enhanced under stressful circumstances. In addition to this normal form of tremor, there are several pathologic tremors that are generally categorized as resting tremor, action tremor, and intention tremor. Action tremor is the most prevalent of these types.

Resting tremor occurs while the limb is relaxed, stationary, and supported against gravity. The amplitude increases during mental stress such as counting backwards and with general movement such as walking. Resting tremor diminishes with target-directed movement such as the finger-to-nose test.

Action tremor occurs during sustained extension of the arm or during voluntary motion such as writing or pouring. The differential diagnosis of an action tremor includes essential tremor, enhanced physiologic tremor, Parkinson's disease, adult-onset idiopathic dystonia, and Wilson's disease. Essential tremor is a visible tremor that occurs when the affected body part maintains position against gravity. It is the most common movement disorder worldwide and has a bimodal age distribution in the teens and 50s. Parkinson's disease is 20 times less common than essential tremor yet affects approximately one million Americans. Initial symptoms include resting tremor beginning in one arm, typically as a flexion–extension elbow movement, a pronation–supination of the forearm, or a pill-rolling finger movement. This tremor worsens with stress and diminishes with voluntary movement. Other signs of Parkinson's disease include rigidity, bradykinesia, impaired postural reflexes, and masked facies.

Intention tremor is a coarse terminal tremor that occurs during visually guided movements as the limb approaches a target. There is significant amplitude fluctuation as the target is approached.

Drug-induced tremor should be differentiated from other forms of tremor. First, other medical causes of tremor such as hyperthyroidism and hypoglycemia should be ruled out. Factors that suggest drug-induced tremor include a temporal relation to the start of therapy with the drug, a dose-response relation, and a lack of tremor progression. Additionally, drug-induced tremor is symmetric for most drugs, except in the setting of drug-induced parkinsonism, in which patients commonly develop unilateral resting tremor. Older age places the patient at higher risk for drug-induced tremor.

Cerebellar tremor presents as unilateral or bilateral, low-frequency intention tremor caused by multiple sclerosis, stroke, or brainstem tumor. Finger-to-nose, finger-to-finger, and heel-to-shin testing results in worsening tremor as the extremity approaches its target. The patient may also have abnormalities of speech, gait, and ocular movements.

Psychogenic tremor is occasionally a consideration in the differential diagnosis of tremor. Psychogenic mimicking is usually diagnosed by distracting the patient with other motor or cognitive tasks. Psychogenic tremor decreases or stops with distraction while organic tremor stays the same or increases.

Medications Associated with Tremor

Amiodarone

Amitriptyline

Amphotericin B

Beta-agonists

Calcitonin

Carbamazepine

Cimetidine

Co-trimoxazole

Cyclosporine

Cytarabine

Epinephrine

Haloperidol

Hypoglycemic agents

Ifosfamide

Interferon-alfa

Lithium

Medroxyprogesterone

Methylphenidate

Metoclopramide

Mexiletine

Procainamide

Pseudoephedrine

Reserpine

Salbutamol

Salmeterol

Selective serotonin reuptake inhibitors

Tacrolimus

Tamoxifen

Terbutaline

Thalidomide

Theophylline

Thioridazine

Thyroxine

Tricyclic antidepressants

Valproic acid

Vidarabine

Causes of Tremor

Action tremor

- Adult-onset idiopathic dystonia
- Enhanced physiologic tremor
- Essential tremor
- Parkinson's disease
- Wilson's disease

Alcohol abuse

Caffeine

Cerebellar lesion

- Multiple sclerosis
- Stroke
- Traumatic brain injury

Cortical tremor

Drug withdrawal

Drugs of abuse

- Amphetamines
- Cocaine
- MDMA
- Nicotine

Intention tremor

Isolated chin tremor

Isolated voice tremor

Medications

Metabolic disorders

- Vitamin B_{12} deficiency
- Hyperparathyroidism
- Hyperthyroidism
- Hypocalcemia
- Hypoglycemia
- Hyponatremia

- Liver disease
- Renal disease
- Wilson's disease

Movement disorders

Neuropathic tremor

Orthostatic tremor

Physiologic tremor

Psychogenic tremor

Resting tremor

Rubral or midbrain tremor

Withdrawal from alcohol, benzodiazepines, or cocaine

Key Historical Features

✓ Age at onset

✓ Exacerbating and relieving factors

✓ Functional limitations

✓ Type of tremor

✓ Rate of progression of the tremor

✓ Past medical history

✓ Medications

✓ Family history

✓ Social history

- Alcohol use
- Caffeine
- Illicit drug use
- Tobacco use

✓ Review of systems

- Diarrhea or weight loss to suggest hyperthyroidism
- Sensation of muscles in the hand or neck being pulled or twisted to suggest dystonia
- Depressive symptoms, cognitive impairment, or other involuntary movements to suggest Wilson's disease

Key Physical Findings

✓ Characteristics of the tremor

- Amplitude

- Frequency
- Affected body part
- Proximal or distal location

✓ Observation of the patient at rest seated in a chair

✓ Observation of the patient performing maneuvers with the arms outstretched in front of the body to evaluate for postural tremor

✓ Observation of the patient performing the finger-to-nose movement to evaluate for an intention tremor

✓ Observation of the patient drinking from a glass, writing, or drawing a rhythmic pattern such as a spiral

✓ Evaluation for rigidity and bradykinesia by flexing and extending the patient's arms

✓ Observation of the patient standing and walking to evaluate for difficulty initiating movement, decreased arm swing, or shuffling gait that may indicate Parkinson's disease

✓ Evaluation for nystagmus

✓ General examination for signs of alcoholism such as spider angiomata or an enlarged liver

✓ Head and neck examination for exophthalmos or thyroid enlargement

✓ Cardiac examination for tachycardia

✓ Neurologic examination for brisk reflexes that may suggest thyrotoxicosis or other abnormalities that may suggest multiple sclerosis

✓ Slit lamp examination for Kayser–Fleischer rings if Wilson's disease is suspected

Suggested Work-Up

Serum glucose	To evaluate for hypoglycemia
Serum electrolytes	To evaluate for hyponatremia
Serum BUN and creatinine	To evaluate for renal disease
Thyroid function tests	To evaluate for thyrotoxicosis
Liver function tests	To evaluate for liver disease

| Serum ceruloplasmin level | In any patient with action tremor who is younger than 40 years of age to evaluate for Wilson's disease. The level is <20 mg/dL in 95% of patients with Wilson's disease |

Additional Work-Up

CT scan or MRI	If cerebellar tumor or stroke is suspected
MRI and cerebrospinal fluid examination of oligoclonal IgG bands	If multiple sclerosis is suspected
Lithium level	If lithium toxicity is suspected

Further reading

Louis ED. Essential tremor. New England Journal of Medicine 2001;345: 887–891.
Morgan JC, Sethi KD. Drug-induced tremors. Lancet Neurology 2005;4: 866–876.
Pahwa R, Lyons KE. Essential tremor: differential diagnosis and current therapy. American Journal of Medicine 2003;115: 134–142.
Smaga S. Tremor. American Family Physician 2003;68: 1545–1552.
Velickovic M, Gracies JM. Movement disorders: keys to identifying and treating tremor. Geriatrics 2002;57: 32–36.

General Discussion

Urinary incontinence is caused by disturbance in the storage function, and occasionally in the emptying function, of the lower urinary tract. A continent sphincter mechanism requires proper angulation between the urethra and the bladder, as well as proper positioning of the urethra so that increases in intra-abdominal pressure are effectively transmitted to the urethra.

Women may undergo an anatomical or neuromuscular injury during childbirth but remain clinically asymptomatic as long as there is compensation by other components of the continence mechanism. Incontinence may not present in a woman until she loses a small percentage of muscle strength and innervation to the urethral sphincter due to aging or other injuries.

Stress incontinence is the involuntary loss of urine during an increase of intra-abdominal pressure. Stress urinary incontinence arises when bladder pressure exceeds urethral pressure during activities such as coughing, laughing, or exercising. The underlying abnormality is typically urethral hypermobility caused by a failure of the normal anatomic supports of the bladder neck. Intrinsic urethral sphincter deficiency, the lack of normal intrinsic pressure within the urethra, may also lead to stress incontinence.

Overactive bladder, also known as urge incontinence, is the involuntary loss of urine preceded by a strong urge to void whether or not the bladder is full. Urge incontinence results from bladder contractions that overwhelm the ability of the cerebral centers to inhibit them. This bladder oversensitivity may originate from the bladder epithelium or detrusor muscle as the result of altered neural activation in the voiding cycle.

Overflow incontinence is urine loss associated with overdistention of the bladder, typically caused by an underactive detrusor muscle and/or outlet obstruction. Patients may present with frequent or constant dribbling, overactive bladder, or stress incontinence. Causes of detrusor muscle underactivity are outlined below. Overflow incontinence is relatively uncommon but is more common in men because of the prevalence of obstructive prostate gland enlargement.

The first goal of the evaluation of urinary incontinence is to identify reversible causes of incontinence so that effective treatments may be instituted. The second goal is to identify conditions that may require special evaluation or referral to a urologist or urogynecologist. Once transient causes and indications for specialty evaluation or referral have been excluded, the third goal is to decide if the patient's symptoms are more suggestive of urge incontinence or stress incontinence. After this has been determined, treatment may be initiated accordingly. If the treatment is ineffective, specialty evaluation may be indicated.

Indications for special evaluation or referral detected by history include the following: recent onset within 2 months of urge incontinence or irritative bladder symptoms, previous surgery for incontinence, previous radical pelvic surgery, or incontinence associated with recurrent symptomatic urinary infections. Physical findings that usually require specialty referral include prostate nodules or asymmetry, gross pelvic prolapse, and neurologic abnormalities suggesting a systemic disorder or spinal cord lesion. Hematuria without infection and significant persistent proteinuria on urinalysis require additional evaluation. Other situations that may require special evaluation or referral are an abnormal postvoid residual volume, treatment failure, consideration of surgical intervention, or an inability to arrive at a presumptive diagnosis and treatment plan.

Medications Associated with Urinary Incontinence

Alpha-adrenergic agonists

Alpha-adrenergic blockers

Angiotensin-converting enzyme (ACE) inhibitors

Anticholinergic agents

Antidepressants

Antihistamines

Antipsychotics

Beta-blockers

Calcium channel blockers

Diuretics

Lithium

Narcotics

Sedatives

Causes of Urinary Incontinence

Overflow incontinence

- Diabetic neuropathy
- Fecal impaction
- Medications
- Prostatic enlargement
- Radiation
- Tumor
- Surgery
- Urethral stricture

Stress incontinence
- Intrinsic sphincter deficiency
- Medications
- Pelvic prolapse
- Radiation damage
- Surgical trauma
- Urethral hypermobility

Urge incontinence
- Alcohol
- Atrophic vaginitis
- Caffeine
- Calculi
- Dementia
- Encephalopathy
- Hypoxemia
- Impaired mobility
- Infection
- Malignancy
- Medications
- Parkinson's disease
- Stroke

Key Historical Features

✓ Frequency of episodes

✓ Degree of bother

✓ Leakage of urine with coughing, laughing, lifting, or sneezing

✓ Leakage of urine associated with a strong urge to urinate

✓ Leakage of urine during sex

✓ Use of pad to protect from leaking urine

✓ Leakage of urine without the patient being aware of the leakage

✓ Time of day or night

✓ Relation to medication treatments

✓ Fluid intake

✓ Voiding habits

✓ How often sleep is interrupted by the need to urinate

✓ Presence of dysuria

✓ Presence of the sensation of incomplete bladder emptying

✓ Frequency of bowel movements

✓ Splinting of the vagina or perineum during defecation

✓ Presence of fecal incontinence

✓ Past medical history

  • Chronic lung disease

  • Cognitive impairment

  • Diabetes

  • Fecal impaction

  • Lumbar disk disease

  • Stroke

✓ Obstetric and gynecological history

  • Gravity and parity

  • Number of vaginal, instrument-assisted, and cesarean deliveries

  • Estrogen status

  • Time interval between deliveries

  • Hysterectomy, vaginal surgery

  • Bladder surgery

  • Pelvic trauma

  • Pelvic radiotherapy

✓ Past surgical history

✓ Medications

Key Physical Findings

✓ General examination for mobility status

✓ Neurologic examination for cognitive status, upper motor neuron lesions such as multiple sclerosis or Parkinson's disease, lower motor neuron lesions such as sacral-nerve root lesions. The lumbosacral nerve roots should be assessed by checking deep tendon reflexes, lower extremity strength, and sharp/dull sensation

✓ Cardiovascular and pulmonary examination to assess for causes of cough

✓ Abdominal examination for masses, diastasis recti, ascites, or organomegaly

✓ Pelvic examination for pelvic masses, organ prolapse, or vaginal atrophy. The levator ani muscle function can be evaluated by asking the patient to tighten her vaginal muscles and hold the contraction as long as possible. The bulbocavernous and clitoral sacral reflexes should be evaluated. The examination should also include an evaluation for inflammation, infection, and atrophy

✓ Rectal examination to evaluate for sphincter tone, fecal impaction, rectal lesions, prostate nodules, prostate asymmetry, or the presence of occult blood

✓ Extremity examination for peripheral edema

✓ Urine leakage should be assessed with coughing or Valsalva in both the supine and standing position.

Suggested Work-Up

Urinalysis	To evaluate for urinary tract infection or diabetes-induced glycosuria
Urine culture	Not routinely indicated but may be useful in identifying the causative organism of infections and in guiding antibiotic therapy
Assessment of postvoid residual volume by catheterization or ultrasonography	To detect urinary retention
	Less than 50 mL is normal, while more than 200 mL is abnormal
Cystometry	To measure bladder pressure during filling, which provides information about bladder capacity and the ability to inhibit detrusor contractions
Cystoscopy	Indicated for the evaluation of patients with incontinence who also have any of the following:

• Hematuria or pyuria
• Irritative voiding symptoms such as frequency, urgency, and urge incontinence in the absence of reversible causes
• Bladder pain

- Recurrent cystitis
- Suburethral mass
- When urodynamic testing fails to duplicate symptoms of urinary incontinence

Additional Work-Up

Cystometric testing	Indicated as part of the evaluation of more complex disorders of bladder filling and voiding, such as the presence of neurologic disease and other comorbid conditions. There is only limited data suggesting its need in the routine evaluation of women with urinary incontinence
Urodynamic testing	May be indicated when surgical treatment of stress incontinence is planned
Pressure-flow voiding studies, uroflometry, and electromyography of the anal sphincter	May be indicated for the assessment of complex and neurogenic causes of urinary incontinence and voiding disorders

Further reading

Culligan PJ, Heit M. Urinary incontinence in women: evaluation and management. American Family Physician 2000;62: 2433–2444.

Morantz CA. ACOG guidelines on urinary incontinence in women. American Family Physician 2005;72: 175.

Norton P, Brubaker L. Urinary incontinence in women. Lancet 2006;367: 57–67.

Wein AJ, Rackley RR. Overactive bladder: a better understanding of pathophysiology, diagnosis, and management. Journal of Urology 2006;175: S5–S10.

Weiss, BD. Diagnostic evaluation of urinary incontinence in geriatric patients. American Family Physician 1998;57: 2675–2684.

General Discussion

Clinically significant weight loss can be defined as the loss of 10 pounds or more than 5% of the usual body weight over 6 to 12 months, especially when the weight loss is progressive. Weight loss greater than 10% represents protein-energy malnutrition, which is associated with impaired physiologic function such as impaired cell-mediated and humoral immunity. Weight loss greater than 20% represents severe protein-energy malnutrition and is associated with organ dysfunction.

Dieting and eating disorders, such as anorexia nervosa and bulimia nervosa, explain most cases of intentional weight loss. Unintentional weight loss can be divided into four problems: anorexia, dysphagia, weight loss despite normal intake, or socioeconomic problems.

Malignancies account for approximately one-third of all patients presenting with unintentional weight loss. Gastrointestinal disorders are the most common nonmalignant organic etiologies in patients with unintentional weight loss, accounting for about 15% of cases. Medications are a frequently overlooked potential etiology of unintentional weight loss, particularly in elderly patients. Adverse effects of medications, such as anorexia, nausea, diarrhea, dysphagia, and dysgeusia may alter the intake, absorption, and utilization of nutrients.

Weight loss occurs commonly in elderly individuals. Among the noninstitutionalized elderly, depression, cancer, and benign gastrointestinal tract diseases are the most common causes of weight loss. Among nursing home residents, psychiatric and neurologic illnesses account for the greatest proportion of weight loss.

In most patients, the etiology of unintentional weight loss may be identified through a detailed history and physical examination. The first step in evaluating a complaint of weight loss is quantifying the weight loss. The symptoms acquired from the history can guide the clinician to one of the four causal categories: anorexia, dysphagia, weight loss despite normal intake, and social factors. The suggested laboratory evaluation is outlined below. Additional testing should be directed by findings on history, physical examination, or initial laboratory evaluation. Patients with normal physical and laboratory findings are unlikely to have a serious physical illness.

Medications Associated with Weight Loss

ACE inhibitors

Alendronate

Allopurinol

Amantadine

Amphetamines

Antibiotics

- Atovaquone
- Ciprofloxacin
- Clarithromycin
- Doxycycline
- Ethambutol
- Griseofulvin
- Metronidazole
- Ofloxacin
- Pentamidine
- Rifabutin
- Tetracycline

Anticholinergics

Anticonvulsants

Antihistamines

Benzodiazepines

Bisphosphonates

Calcium-channel blockers

Carbamazepine

Chemotherapeutic agents

Clonidine

Corticosteroids

Decongestants

Digoxin

Dopamine agonists

Gold

Hormone replacement therapy

Hydralazine

Hydrochlorothiazide

Iron

Levodopa

Lithium

Metformin

Methimazole

Neuroleptics

Nicotine

Nitroglycerin

NSAIDs

Opiates

Penicillamine

Pergolide

Phenytoin

Potassium

Propranolol

Quinidine

SSRIs

Selegiline

Spironolactone

Statins

Theophylline

Tricyclic antidepressants

Causes of Weight Loss

Alcoholism

Cardiovascular disease

- Congestive heart failure
- Mesenteric ischemia

Cocaine use

Dietary factors (low-salt, low-cholesterol diets)

Endocrine disorders

- Adrenal insufficiency
- Diabetes mellitus
- Hyperparathyroidism
- Hyperthyroidism
- Hypothyroidism
- Panhypopituitarism
- Pheochromocytoma

Gastrointestinal disease

- Atrophic gastritis
- Celiac disease
- Cholelithiasis
- Chronic pancreatitis
- Constipation
- Diarrhea
- Dysphagia (oropharyngeal or esophageal)

- Gastroparesis
- Inflammatory bowel disease
- Malabsorption due to bacterial overgrowth, pancreatic exocrine deficiency, or celiac disease
- Peptic ulcer disease
- Pseudo-obstruction
- Reflux esophagitis

Inability to feed self

Infections

- Fungal disease
- HIV infection
- Parasites
- Subacute bacterial endocarditis
- Tuberculosis

Malignancies

- Breast
- Gastrointestinal
- Genitourinary
- Hepatobiliary
- Hematologic
- Lung
- Ovarian
- Prostate

Medications

Neurologic disease

- Cerebrovascular accident
- Delirium
- Dementia
- Multiple sclerosis
- Parkinson's disease
- Quadriplegia
- Tardive dyskinesia

Nutritional disorders

Oral factors

- Periodontal disease
- Poor dentition
- Xerostomia

Pulmonary disease
- Chronic obstructive pulmonary disease

Psychiatric disorders
- Anorexia nervosa
- Anxiety disorders
- Depression
- Paranoia

Renal disease
- Hemodialysis
- Nephrotic syndrome
- Uremia

Rheumatologic disease
- Giant cell arteritis
- Scleroderma

Socioeconomic conditions

Swallowing disorders

Visual impairments

Key Historical Features

✓ Amount of weight loss

✓ Determine if the patient is predominantly not hungry, is feeling nauseated after meals, is having difficulty eating or swallowing, or is having functional or social problems that may be interfering with the ability to obtain or enjoy food

✓ Presence of indigestion or reflux symptoms

✓ Abdominal pain

✓ Changes in bowel habits

✓ In geriatric patients, interview a knowledgeable caretaker

✓ Dietary history
- Availability of food
- Use of nutritional or herbal supplements
- Amount of food consumed
- Adequacy of the patient's diet
- Daily caloric intake

✓ Discussion of functional and mental status

✓ Past medical history, especially previous gastrointestinal conditions

✓ Past surgical history, especially previous gastrointestinal surgery

✓ Medications

✓ Social history

- Financial situation
- Lifestyle
- Living arrangements/home environment
- Occupation
- Support network
- Travel
- Use of transportation

✓ Thorough review of systems

Key Physical Findings

✓ Vital signs

✓ Height, weight, and body mass index

✓ Examination of the oral cavity

✓ Cardiopulmonary examination

✓ Abdominal examination

✓ Rectal examination

✓ Mental status examination and formal cognitive testing with an instrument such as the Folstein Mini-Mental State Exam

✓ Evaluation for depression using an instrument such as the PHQ-9 or the Geriatric Depression Scale

✓ Examination of the nervous system

✓ Functional assessment, including evaluations of sight, hearing, gait, and self-care ability (tools include the Katz scale of activities of daily living and the Lawton scale of instrumental activities of daily living)

Suggested Work-Up

CBC	To evaluate for infection, anemia, or lymphoproliferative disorder
Chemistry panel	To evaluate for diabetes mellitus, dehydration, or renal dysfunction
Thyroid stimulating hormone	To evaluate for hypo- or hyperthyroidism

Urinalysis	To evaluate for infection, renal dysfunction, or dehydration
Fecal occult blood test	To screen for gastrointestinal malignancy
Chest x-ray	To evaluate for infection, malignancy, or cardiopulmonary disease
Upper endoscopy or upper GI series	Should be considered in patients with anorexia, absence of other symptoms, and persistent weight loss because peptic ulcer disease and gastroesophageal reflux may be silent

Additional Work-Up

Erythrocyte sedimentation rate	To evaluate for inflammation
Blood culture	If infection is suspected
PPD	If tuberculosis is suspected
HIV test	If risk factors are present for HIV infection is suspected
RPR	If risk factors for syphilis are present or physical findings suggest the presence of syphilis infection
Growth hormone	To evaluate for endocrine deficiency
Testosterone level	To evaluate for low testosterone levels
Sigmoidoscopy or colonoscopy	If a colonic lesion is suspected
CT scanning	Low yield but may be helpful in diagnosing malignancy, abscess, chronic pancreatitis, intestinal complications, etc.
Serum prealbumin, transferrin, and albumin	Not useful in determining the etiology of weight loss, but may be used to guide supplement selection

Further reading

Alibhai SM, Greenwood C, Payette H. An approach to the management of unintentional
     weight loss in elderly people. Canadian Medical Association Journal 2005;172: 773–780.
Bouras EP, Lange SM, Scolapio JS. Rational approach to patients with unintentional weight loss.
     Mayo Clinic Proceedings 2001;76: 923–929.
Gazewood JD, Mehr DR. Diagnosis and management of weight loss in the elderly. Journal of
     Family Practice 1998;47: 19–25.
Huffman GB. Evaluating and treating unintentional weight loss in the elderly. American Family
     Physician 2002;65: 640–650.
Robertson RG, Montagnini M. Geriatric failure to thrive. American Family Physician
     2004;70:343–350.

Index